AF797389

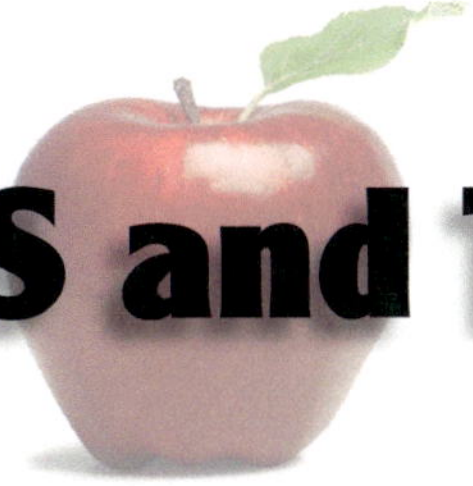

To PARENTS and TEACHERS

Children are constantly barraged with confusing messages about how to eat, what to drink, and how to care for their God-given bodies. This book teaches children how to properly care for their bodies by presenting simple and sound principles of healthy living and nutrition.

This book is adapted from the *First Book in Physiology and Hygiene,,* by John Harvey Kellogg, M.D. Dr. Kellogg's teachings on health were revolutionary in 1887, when the book was first published. Well into the twentieth century people from around the world, celebrities and dignitaries alike, visited Battle Creek Sanitarium in Battle Creek, Michigan, to learn principles of healthy living from Dr. Kellogg himself. Even today, with advances in science and medicine occurring daily, healthcare professionals continue to teach and use many of Dr. Kellogg's methods.

The goals of Dr. Kellogg's original book remain central to this latest version:

1. To present as fully as possible and proper in a work of this type a statement of the laws of healthful living, giving special attention to the subject of stimulants and narcotics.

2. To present in a simple manner such anatomical and physiological facts as shall give the child a good fundamental knowledge of the structure and functions of the human body.

3. To present each topic in such clear and simple language as to enable the pupil to comprehend the subject-matter with little aid from the parent or teacher; and to observe in the manner of presentation the principle that the things to be studied should be placed before the mind of the child before they are named. A natural and logical order has been observed in the sequence of topics. Technical terms have been used very sparingly, and only in their natural order, and are then fully explained and their pronunciation indicated, so that it is not thought necessary to append a glossary.

4. To present the subjects of Physiology and Hygiene in the light of the most recent authentic researches in these branches of science, and to avoid the numerous errors which have for many years been current in the school literature of these subjects.

DISCLAIMER

The content of the this book is provided for general information only and is not intended in any way to substitute for professional medical advice. The content is not intended to be relied upon for medical diagnosis or treatment. Always seek the advice of a physician or other qualified health professional for any health concern. It is the responsibility of the teacher, parent or reader to research the accuracy, completeness, and usefulness of all information provided in this book, and to consult with a professional health care provider as to whether the information can benefit them. Neither the author, editor, publisher nor the endorsers of this book assume responsibility or liability for any consequence resulting directly or indirectly for any action or inaction taken based on or made in reliance on the information contained in this book, neither are they liable for any damage or loss related to the accuracy, completeness or timeliness of any information contained in this book. Since medical developments occur daily, this book may contain outdated material. While the author, editor, and publisher make every reasonable effort to present current and accurate information, no guarantee of any kind is made.

The writings of the original authors referenced in this book have been edited to use current terminology and to reflect modern practices, while retaining the authors' original intent.

A WORD from MRS. WHITE

Body and soul belong to God. He gave his Son for the redemption of the world, and because of this, we have been granted a new lease of life, a limited time in which to develop characters of perfect loyalty. God has redeemed us from the slavery of sin, and has made it possible for us to live renewed, transformed lives of service.

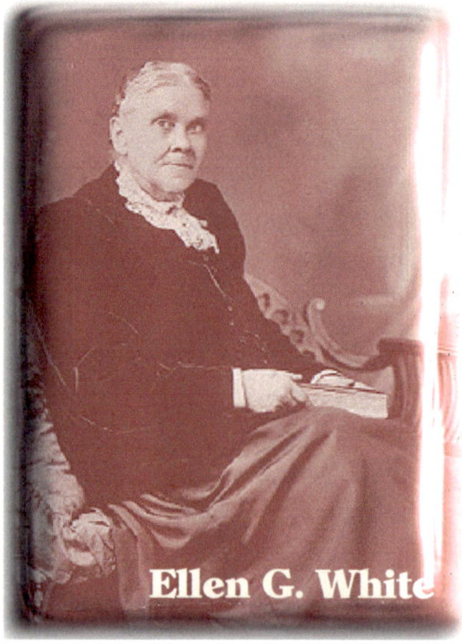

God's stamp is upon us. He has bought us, and he desires us to remember that our physical, mental, and moral powers belong to him. Time and influence, reason, affection, and conscience,--all are God's, and are to be used only in harmony with his will. They are not to be used in accordance with the direction of the world; for the world is under a leader who is at enmity with God.

The flesh, the house of our soul, belongs to God. Every sinew, every muscle, is his. In no case are we by neglect or abuse to weaken a single organ. We are to cooperate with God by keeping the body in the very best possible condition of health, that it may be a temple where the Holy Spirit may abide, molding, according to the will of God, every physical and spiritual power.

The mind must be stored with pure principles. Truth must be graven on the tablets of the soul. The memory must be filled with the precious truths of the Word. Then, like beautiful gems, these truths will flash out in the life.

The value that God places on the work of his hands, the love he has for his children, is revealed by the gift he made to redeem men. Adam fell under the dominion of Satan. He brought sin into the world, and death by sin. God gave his only begotten Son to save man. This he did that he might be just, and yet the justifier of all who accept Christ. Man sold himself to Satan, but Jesus bought back the race.

At an infinite cost to heaven we have been given a second probation. Then should not God be in all our thoughts? Should not his will control our actions?

. . .We, and all that we have, belong to God. We should not regard it as a sacrifice to give him the affection of our hearts. The heart itself should be given to him as a willing offering.

Impressed with man's great obligation to God, Paul wrote: "I beseech you therefore, brethren, by the mercies of God, that ye present your bodies a living sacrifice, holy, acceptable unto God, which is your reasonable service." He urges a recognition of God's claims. "Know ye not," he asks, "that your body is the temple of the Holy Spirit which is in you, which ye have of God, and ye are not your own? For ye are bought with a price: therefore glorify God in your body, and in your spirit, which are God's."

Ellen G. White
Youth's Instructor
November 8, 1900

DR. JOHN HARVEY KELLOGG'S

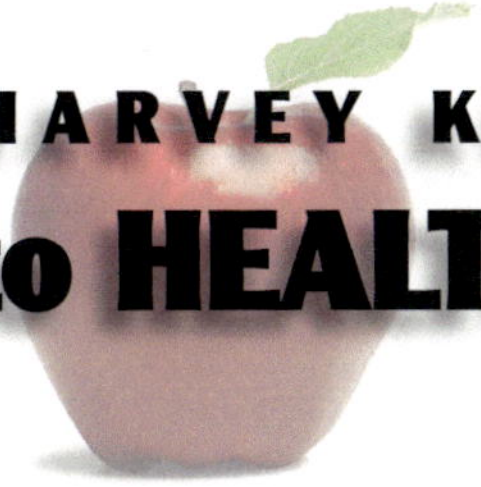

CHILD'S GUIDE to HEALTH and HYGIENE

Mustard Seed Imprints™
Clackamas, Oregon
www.MustardSeedImprints.com

DR. JOHN HARVEY KELLOGG'S
CHILD'S GUIDE TO HEALTH AND HYGIENE

Mustard Seed Imprints
P.O. Box 1211
Clackamas, Oregon 97015

orders@MustardSeedImprints.com; http://www.MustardSeedImprints.com

All rights reserved. No part of this book may be used or reproduced or transmitted in any form or by any means, electronic or mechanical, including photocopying, recording, by any information storage or retrieval system without prior written permission of the publisher except in the case of brief quotations embodied in critical articles and reviews. Making copies of any part of this book for any purpose other than your own personal use is a violation of United States copyright laws.

Copyright © 2008 Mustard Seed Imprints

Cover and inside design: Jon D. Beaty
Cover and inside photos © iStockphoto.com

ISBN 978-0-9817475-0-7

CONTENTS

Enhance your child's learning with the companion workbook!

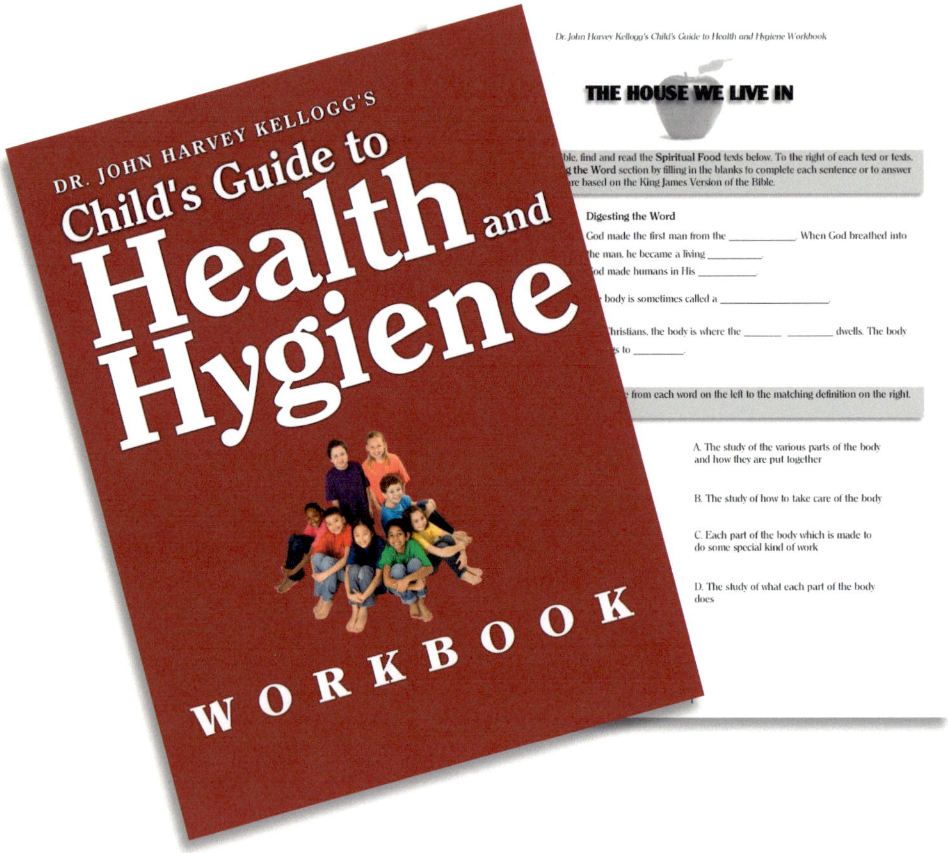

Available at
http://Kellogg.MustardSeedImprints.com

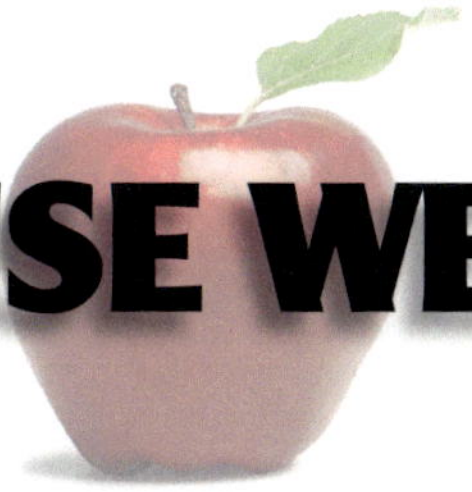

The HOUSE WE LIVE IN

The object of this book is to tell the boys and girls who read it about a wonderful house. You have all seen some very beautiful houses. Perhaps they were made of brick or stone, with fine porches, having around them tall shade trees, smooth lawns, pretty flower-beds, walks, and sparkling fountains. Perhaps some of you live in such a house, or have visited some friend who does. If so, you know that the inside of the house is even more beautiful than the outside. There are elegant chairs and sofas in the rooms, rich carpets and rugs on the floors, fine mirrors and beautiful pictures upon the walls–everything one could wish to have in a house. Do you not think such a house a nice one to live in?

The body is like a house. Each of us has a house of his own which is far more wonderful and more curious than the grandest palace ever built. It is not a very large house. It has just room enough in it for one person. This house, which belongs to each one of us, is called the body.

Do you know what a machine is? People make machines to help them work and to do many useful things. A wheelbarrow or a wagon is a machine to carry loads. A sewing-machine helps to make garments for us to wear. Clocks and watches are machines for keeping time.

A machine has different parts. A wheelbarrow has a box in which to carry things, two handles to hold by, and a wheel for rolling it along. Some machines, like wheelbarrows and wagons, have

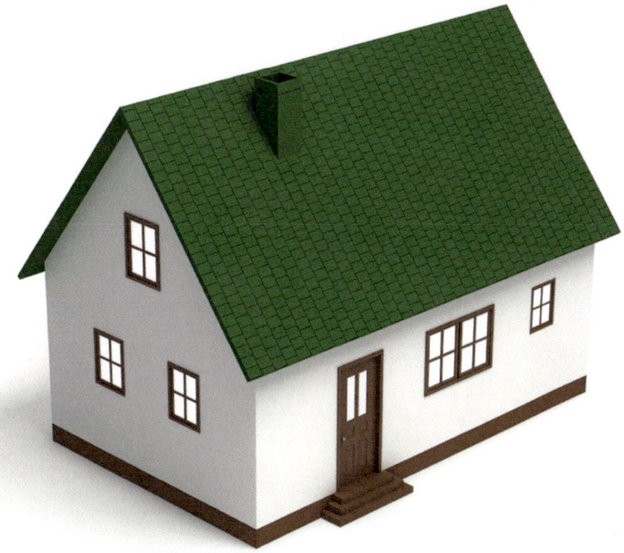

but few parts, and it is very easy for us to learn how they work. But there are other machines, like watches and sewing-machines, which have many different parts, and it is more difficult to learn all about them and what they do.

The body is like a machine. In some ways the body is more like a machine than like a house. It has many different parts which are made to do a great many different kinds of work. We see with our eyes, hear with our ears, walk with our legs and feet, and do a great many things with our hands. If you have ever seen the inside of a watch or a clock you know how many curious little wheels it has. And yet a watch or a clock can do but one thing, and that is to tell us the time of day. The body has a great many more parts than a watch has, and for this reason the body can do many more things than a watch can do. It is more difficult, too, to learn about the body than about a watch.

If we want to know all about a machine and how it works, we must study all its different parts and learn how they are put together, and what each part does. Then, if we want the machine to work well and to last a long time, we must know how to use it and how to take proper care of it. Do you think your watch would keep the time well if you should neglect to wind it, or if you should break any of its wheels?

It is just the same with the human machine which we call the body. We must learn its parts, and what they are for, how they are made, how they are put together, and how they work. Then we must learn how to take proper care of the body, so that its parts will be able to work well and last a long time.

Each part of the body which is made to do some special kind of work is called an organ. The eye, the ear, the nose, a hand, an arm, any part of the body that does something, is an organ.

The study of the various parts of the body and how they are put together is *anatomy* (uh-nat´-o-mee). The study of what each part of the body does is *physiology* (fiz-ee-ol´-o-jee). The study of how to take care of the body is *hygiene* (hy´-jeen).

POINTS TO REMEMBER

1. The body is something like a house. It has an outside and an inside; it has hollow places inside of it, and there are many wonderful things in them.

2. The body is also like a wonderful machine.

3. It is necessary to take good care of the body in order to keep it well and useful, just as we would take good care of a machine to keep it from wearing out too soon.

4. The body has many different parts, called organs, each of which has some particular work to do.

5. In learning about the body, we have to study anatomy, physiology, and hygiene.

6. The study of the various parts of the body, how they are formed and joined together, is anatomy. Physiology tells us what the body does, hygiene tells us how to take care of it.

An OVERVIEW of the BODY

Parts of the Body–What do we call the main part of a tree? The trunk, you say. The main part of the body is also called its trunk. There are two arms and two legs growing out of the human trunk. The branches of a tree we call limbs, and so we speak of the arms and legs as limbs. We sometimes call the arms the upper extremities (ex-trem´-uh-tees), and the legs the lower extremities. At the top of the trunk is the head.

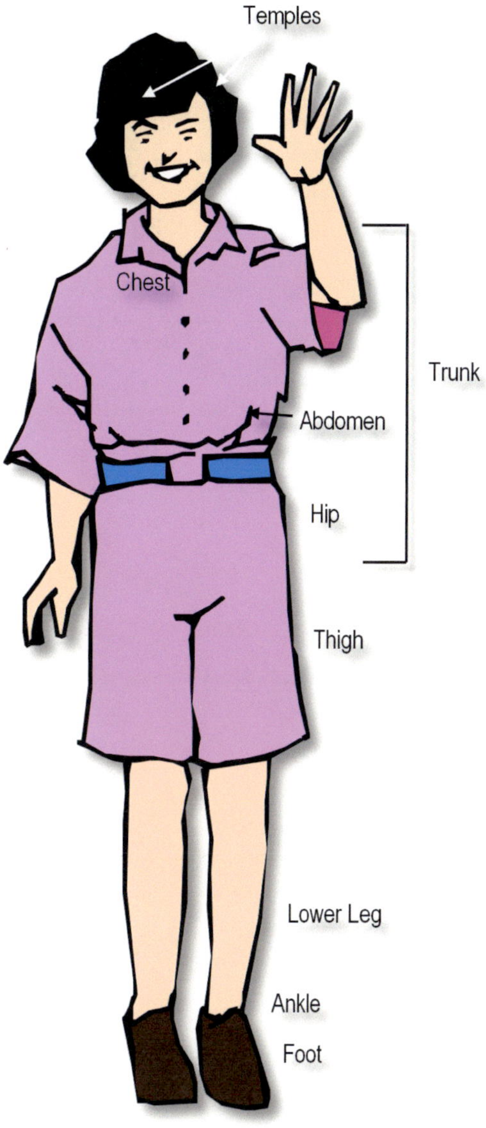

Names of the Parts–Now let us look more closely at these different parts. As we speak the name of each part, touch that part of yourself which is named. We will begin with the head. The chief parts of the head are the skull and the face. The forehead, the temples, the cheeks, the eyes, the ears, the nose, the mouth, and the chin are parts of the face.

The chief parts of the trunk are the chest, the abdomen (ab-duh´-men), and the backbone. The head is joined to the trunk by the neck. Each arm has a shoulder, upper-arm, fore-arm, wrist, and hand. The fingers are a part of the hand.

Each leg has a hip, thigh, lower leg, ankle, and foot. The toes are a part of the foot.

Our hands and face and the whole body are covered with something as soft and smooth as the finest silk. It is the skin. What is it that grows from the skin on the head? and what at the ends of the fingers and the toes? We shall

POINTS TO REMEMBER

1. The body has a head and trunk, two arms, and two legs.

2. The parts of the head are the skull and face. The forehead, temples, cheeks, eyes, ears, nose, mouth and chin are parts of the face.

3. The parts of the trunk are, the chest, abdomen, and backbone. The neck joins the head and trunk.

4. Each arm has a shoulder, upper-arm, forearm, wrist, and hand. The fingers belong to the hand.

5. Each leg has a hip, thigh, lower leg, ankle, and foot. The toes belong to the foot.

6. The whole body is covered by the skin.

7. The two sides of the body are alike.

learn more about the skin, the hair, and the nails in another lesson.

The body has two sides, the right side and the left side, which are alike. We have two eyes, two ears, two arms, etc. We have but one nose, one mouth, and one chin, but each of these organs has two halves, which are just alike.

The INSIDE of the BODY

Thus far we have taken only a brief look at the outside of the body, just as if we had looked at the case of a watch, and of course we have found out very little about its many wonderful parts. Very likely you want to ask a great many questions, such as, *How does the inside of the body look? What is in the skull? What is in the chest? What is in the abdomen? Why do we eat and drink? Why do we become hungry and thirsty? What makes us tired and sleepy? How do we keep warm? Why do we breathe? How do we grow? How do we move about? How do we talk, laugh, and sing? How do we see, hear, feel, taste, and smell? How do we remember, think, and reason?* All these, and a great many more interesting questions, you will find answered in the following lessons, if you study each one well.

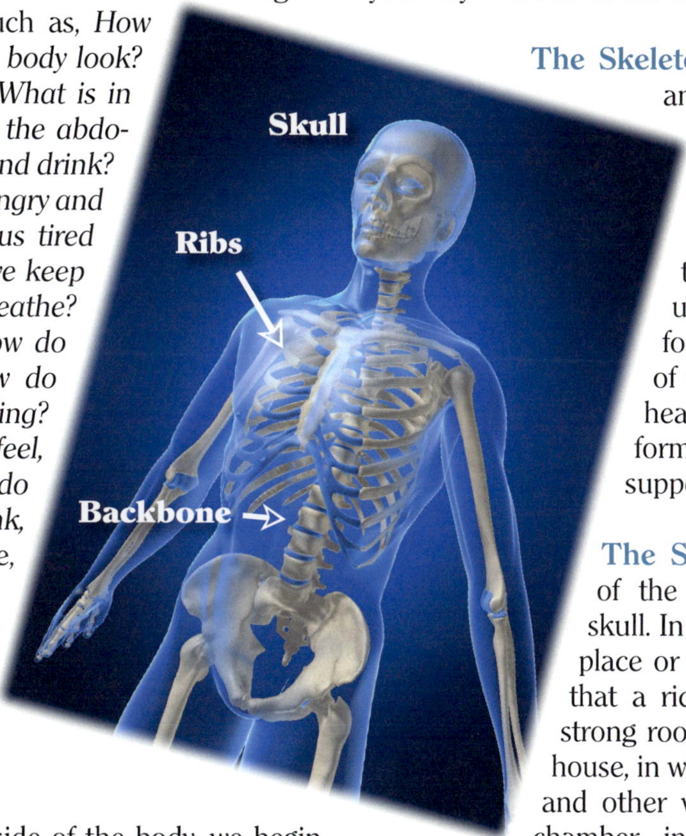

When we study the inside of the body, we begin to understand how wonderfully we are made. We cannot all see the inside of the body, and it is not necessary that we should do so. Many learned men and women have spent their whole lives in seeking to find out all about our bodies and the bodies of various animals.

The Bones–If you take hold of your arm, it seems soft on the outside; and if you press upon it, you will feel something hard inside. The soft part is called flesh. The hard part is called bone. If you wish, you can easily get one of the bones of an animal at the butcher's shop, or you may find one in the fields.

The Skeleton–All the bones of an animal, when placed properly together, have nearly the shape of the body, and are called the skeleton (skel′-uh-ton). The skeleton forms the framework of the body, just as the heavy timbers of a house form its framework. It supports all the parts.

The Skull–The bony part of the head is called the skull. In the skull is a hollow place or chamber. You know that a rich man often has a strong room or box in his fine house, in which to keep his gold and other valuable things. The chamber in the skull is the strongroom of the body. It has strong, tough walls of bone, and contains the brain. The brain is the most important, and also the most tender and delicate organ in the whole body. This is why it is so carefully guarded from injury.

The Backbone–The framework of the back is called the backbone. This is not a single bone, but a row of bones arranged one above another. Each bone has a hole through it, about as large as one of your fingers. A large branch from the brain, called the spinal cord, runs down through the middle of the backbone, so that the separate bones look as if they were strung on the spinal cord, like beads on a string.

The Trunk–The trunk of the body, like the skull, is hollow. Its walls are formed partly by the backbone and the ribs and partly by flesh. A fleshy wall divides the hollow of the trunk into two parts, an upper chamber called the chest, and a lower called the abdomen.

The Lungs and Heart–The chest contains a pair of organs called the lungs, with which we breathe. It also contains something which we can feel beating at the left side. This is the heart. The heart lies between the two lungs, and a little to the left side.

The Stomach and Liver–In the abdomen are some very wonderful organs that do different kinds of work for the body. Among them are the stomach, the bowels, and the liver. There are, also, other organs whose names we shall learn when we come to study them.

Care of the Body–We have only begun to study the beautiful house in which we live, and yet have we not learned enough to show us how great and wise is the Creator who made us and all the wonderful machinery within our bodies? If some one should give you a beautiful present, would you treat it carelessly and spoil it, or would you take good care of it and keep it nice as long as possible? Ought we not to take such care of our bodies as to keep them in that perfect and beautiful condition in which our kind and good Creator gave them to us?

POINTS TO REMEMBER

1. The body has a framework, called the skeleton.

2. The skeleton is made up of many different parts, each of which is called a bone.

3. The bones are covered by the flesh.

4. The bones of the head form the skull, which is hollow and contains the brain.

5. A row of bones arranged in the back, one above another, forms the backbone. The backbone has a canal running through it lengthwise, in which lies the spinal cord.

6. The trunk is hollow, and has two chambers, one called the cavity of the chest, and the other the cavity of the abdomen.

7. The chest contains the two lungs and the heart.

8. The abdomen contains the stomach, liver, and many other very important organs.

9. Is it not our duty to take good care of our bodies as we would of some nice present from a friend?

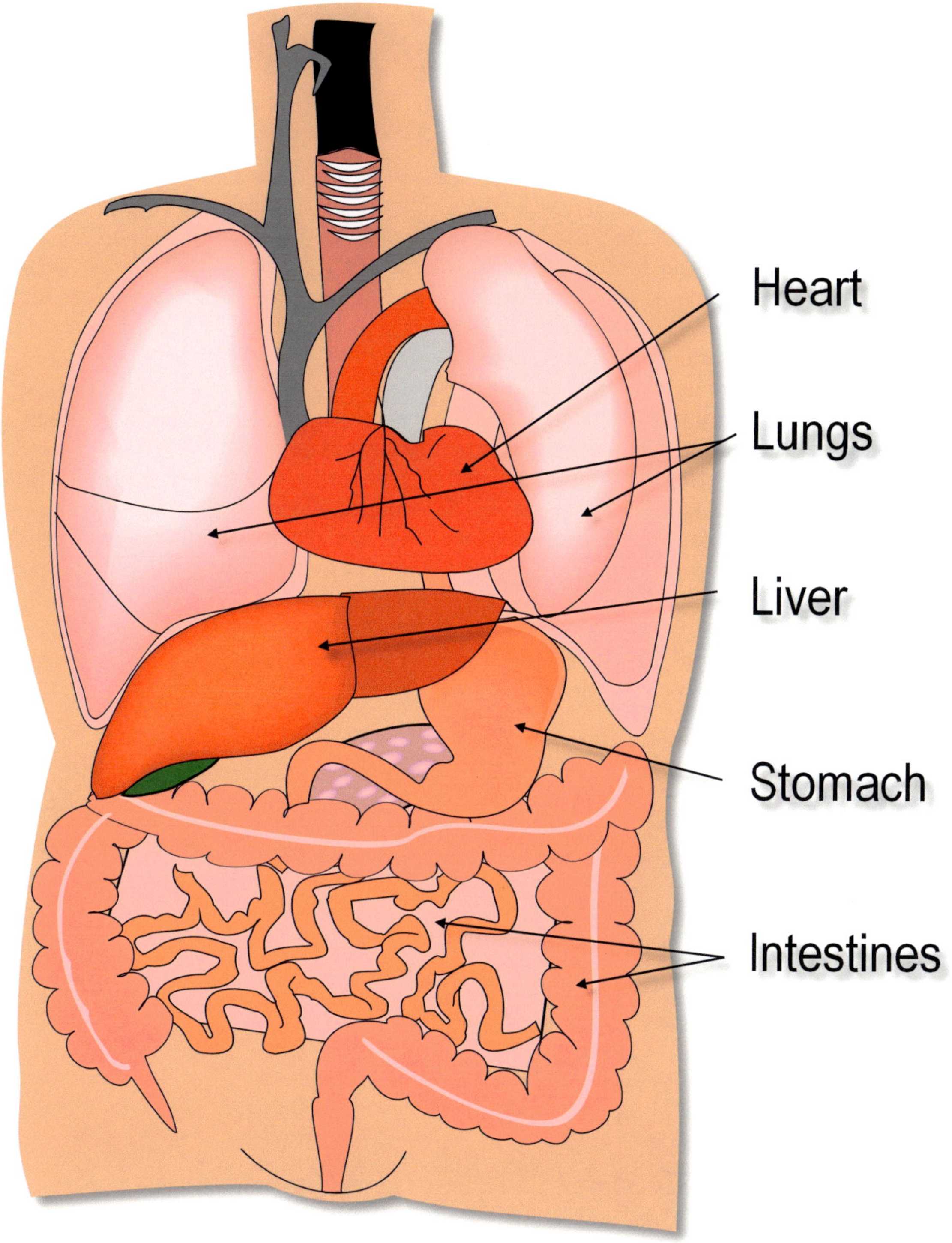
Heart
Lungs
Liver
Stomach
Intestines

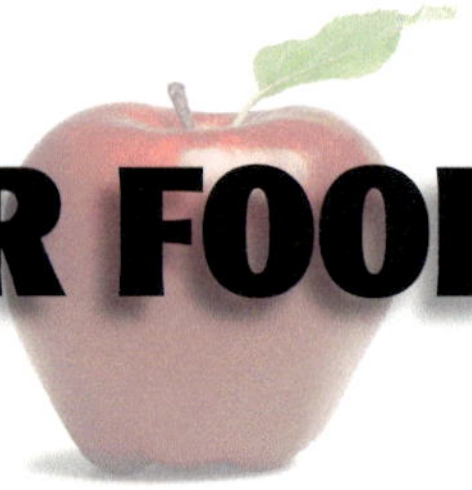

OUR FOODS

We all know very well that if we do not eat we shall rapidly lose in weight, and become very weak and feeble. Did you ever think how much one eats in the course of a lifetime? Let us see if we can figure it up. How much do you suppose a boy eats in a day? Let us say two pounds. How much does he eat in a year? There are three hundred and sixty-five days in a year; 365 multiplied by 2 equals 730. So a boy eats a good many times his own weight in a year. How much would a person eat in fifty years?

Our bodies are composed of what we eat. If we eat bad food, our bodies will be made out of poor material, and will not be able to do their work well. So you see how important it is to learn something about our foods. We ought to know what things are good for us to eat, and what will do us harm.

Foods and Poisons–Foods are those substances which nourish the body and keep it in good working order.

Our foods are obtained from both animals and plants. All food really comes from plants, however, since those animals which we sometimes use as food themselves live upon the vegetables which they eat. For example, the ox and the cow eat grass and furnish us beef and milk. Chickens eat corn and other grains, and supply us with eggs.

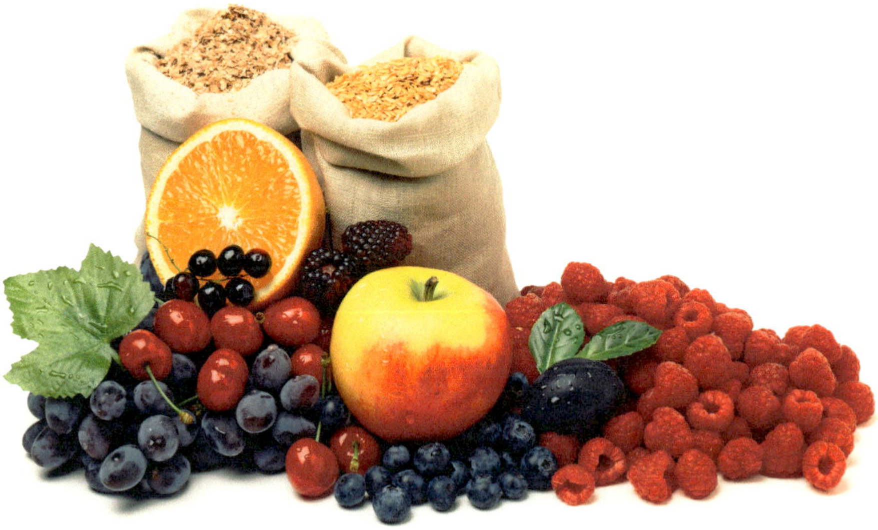

The principal animal foods are milk, cheese, eggs, and the different kinds of flesh–beef, mutton, pork, fish, fowl, and wild game.

We obtain a great many more kinds of food from plants than from animals. Plant foods are the best, and when freshly harvested and in plentiful supply are better for the body than animal foods. Most plant foods are included in three classes–fruits, grains, and vegetables.

Fruits are the fleshy parts of plants which contain the seeds. Our most common fruits are apples, pears, peaches, plums, cherries, and various kinds of nuts. Perhaps you know of some other kinds of fruits besides those mentioned. A parent or teacher will tell you that tomatoes, watermelons, and pumpkins are really fruits, though they are not generally so called.

The seeds of grass-like plants are known as grains, of which we have wheat, rye, barley, corn, and rice. There are a few seeds that grow in pods, such as peas and beans, which somewhat resemble grains.

We eat the leaves, stems, or roots of some plants, as cabbages, celery, turnips, and potatoes. Foods of this kind are called vegetables.

There are other things, which, if we eat or drink them, will make us sick or otherwise do us harm. These are called poisons. Only such food as is pure and free from poisons is good or safe for us to use.

Narcotics and Stimulants–There are a number of substances known as narcotics and stimulants, which, from their effects upon the body, may be classed as poisons. Tobacco, opium, alcohol, and barbiturates (bar·bi´·tu·rates) are included in this class. Death has often been caused by taking small quantities of any of these poisonous drugs. We shall learn more of the effects of tobacco and alcohol in future lessons.

POINTS TO REMEMBER

1. Our bodies are made of what we eat.

2. Things which will help us to grow strong and well, if we eat them, are foods.

3. We get foods from plants and animals.

4. There are several kinds of animal foods, and three classes of plant foods–fruits, grains, and vegetables.

5. Freshly harvested plant foods are the best for our bodies.

6. Things which make us sick when we eat them, are poisons.

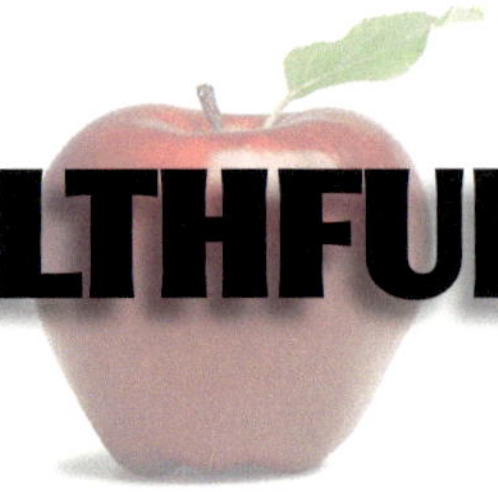

UNHEALTHFUL FOODS

Most persons eat many things which are not good for them. Some people do not stop to think whether what they eat is good for them or likely to do them harm. Sometimes, without knowing it, we eat things which are harmful to us. Do you not think that we should try to learn what is good to eat and what is not good, and then be very careful not to eat anything which is likely to do us harm?

Diseased Foods–When a person is sick, they are said to be diseased. Animals are sometimes sick or diseased. Vegetables are also sometimes diseased. Animals and vegetables that are diseased are not good for food. Dishonest people, however, sometimes sell them to those who do not know that they are unfit to be eaten.

Pork, the flesh of the hog, is more likely to be diseased than any other kind of animal food.

Beef and mutton may be diseased also. Sheep and cattle are sometimes sick of diseases very much like those which human beings have. Meat which is pale, yellowish, or of a dark red color, is unhealthful, and should not be eaten. Meat should never be eaten raw. It should always be well cooked.

Unripe Foods–Most vegetable foods are unfit to be eaten when green or unripe, especially if uncooked. Sometimes persons are made very sick indeed by eating such articles as green apples or unripe peaches.

Stale or Decayed Foods–Food which has been allowed to stand until it is spoiled, or has become stale, musty, or moldy, such as moldy bread or fruit, or tainted meat, is unfit to be eaten, and is often a cause of very severe sickness. Canned fish or other meats spoil very quickly after the cans are opened, and should be eaten the same day.

Adulterated (uh-dul´-ter-ayt-ed) Foods–Many of our foods are sometimes spoiled or injured by persons who put into them cheap substances which are harmful to health. They do this so as to make more money in selling them. This is called adulteration. Foods which are most likely to be adulterated are milk and meat.

Milk is most often adulterated by adding water, though sometimes other things are added. Sometimes the water is not pure, and people are made sick and die. The adulteration of milk or any other food is a very wicked practice.

Meat may be adulterated by mixing other, less expensive or lower quality meats.

Sugar and Syrups–A great deal of the sugar and syrups which we buy is made from corn by a curious process, which changes the starch of the corn into sugar. Sugar which has been made in this way is not so sweet as cane sugar, and is not healthful.

Condiments or Seasonings–These are substances which are added to our food for the purpose of giving to it special flavors. Condiments are not foods, because they do not nourish the body in any way, and are not necessary to preserve it in health.

The most common condiments are, mustard, pepper, pepper-sauce, ginger, cayenne-pepper, and spices. All these substances are irritating. If we put mustard upon the skin, it will make the skin red, and in a little time will raise a blister. If we happen to get a little pepper in the eye, it makes it smart and become very red and inflamed. When we take these things into the stomach, they cause the stomach to smart, and its lining membrane becomes red just as the skin or the eye does.

Nature has put into our foods very nice flavors to make us enjoy eating them. Condiments are likely to do us great harm, and hence it is far better not to use them.

Tobacco–Most of you know that tobacco is obtained from a plant which has long, broad leaves. These leaves are dried and then rolled up into cigarettes, cigars, ground into snuff, or prepared for chewing.

Tobacco has a smarting, sickening taste. Do you think it would be good to eat? Why not?

You know that tobacco makes people sick when they first begin to use it. This is because it contains a very deadly poison, called nicotine (nick´·o·teen).

If you give tobacco to a cat or a dog, it will become very sick. A boy once gave a piece of tobacco to a monkey, which swallowed it not knowing what a bad thing it was. The monkey soon became sick and died.

Many learned doctors have noticed the effects which come from using tobacco, and they all say it does great harm to boys and girls, that it makes them puny and weak, and prevents them from growing up to be strong and useful. If tobacco is not good for children, do you think it can be good for adults? Certainly you will say, *No.*

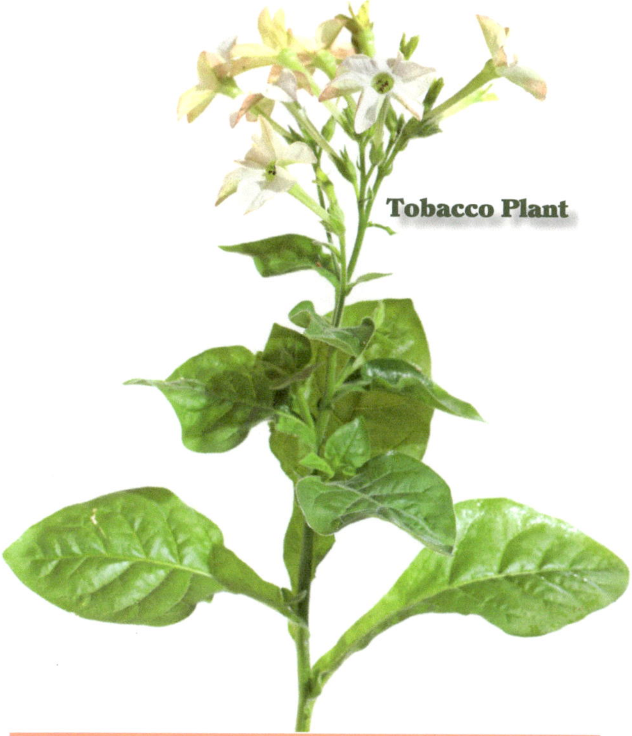

POINTS TO REMEMBER

1. Both animals and plants are sometimes diseased. Flesh obtained from sick or diseased animals is unfit for food.

2. Unripe, stale, and moldy foods are unfit to be eaten and likely to cause severe illness.

3. Foods are sometimes spoiled by having things mixed with them which are not food, or which are poisonous or poor quality. Foods most liable to be adulterated in this way are milk and meat.

4. Tobacco, while not actually eaten, is thought by some persons to be a food, but it is not. It is a poison, and injures all who use it.

5. Children who use tobacco do not grow strong in body and mind.

OUR DRINKS

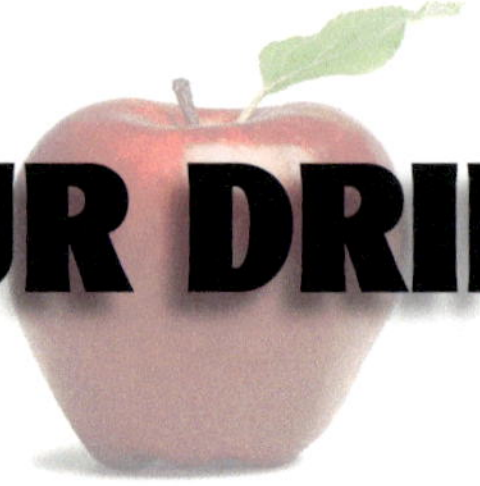

Water is really the only drink. It is the only substance which will satisfy thirst. All other fluids which we drink consist mostly of water. Thus, lemonade is lemon-juice and water. Milk is chiefly water. Wine, beer, cider, and such liquids contain alcohol and many other things, mixed with water.

Why We Need Water–If we should wet a sponge and lay it away, it would become dry in a few hours, as the water would pass off into the air. Our bodies are losing water all the time, and we need to drink to keep ourselves from drying up.

Water is also very necessary for other purposes. It softens our food so that we can chew and swallow it, and helps to carry it around in the body after it has been digested, in a way about which we shall learn in future lessons.

Still another use for water is to dissolve and wash out of our bodies, through the sweat of the skin, and in other ways, the waste and worn-out particles which are no longer of any use.

Impure Water–Most waters have more or less substances dissolved in them. Water which has much lime in it is called *hard water*. Such water is not so good to drink, or for use in cooking, as *soft water*. That water is best which holds no substances in solution. Well-water sometimes contains substances which soak into wells from vaults or cesspools. Slops which are poured upon the ground soak down out of sight; but the foul substances which they contain are not destroyed. They remain in the soil, and when the rains come, they are washed down into the well if it

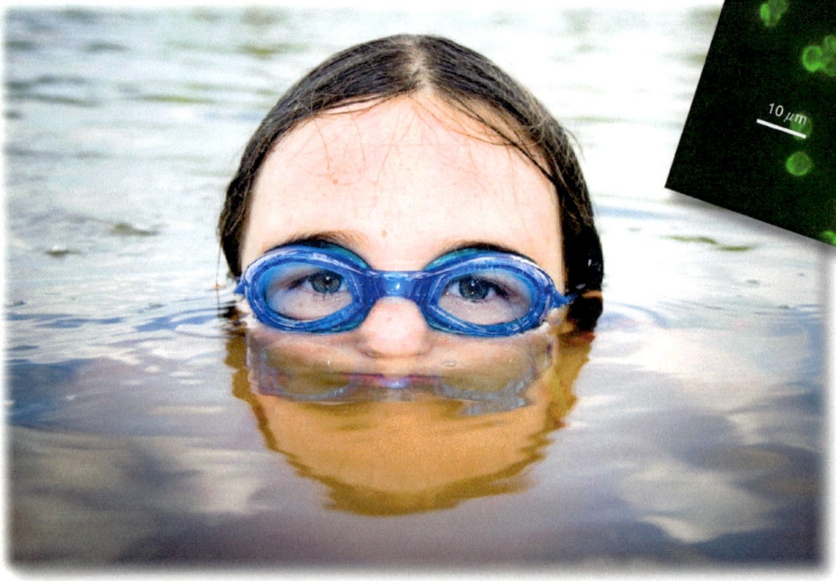

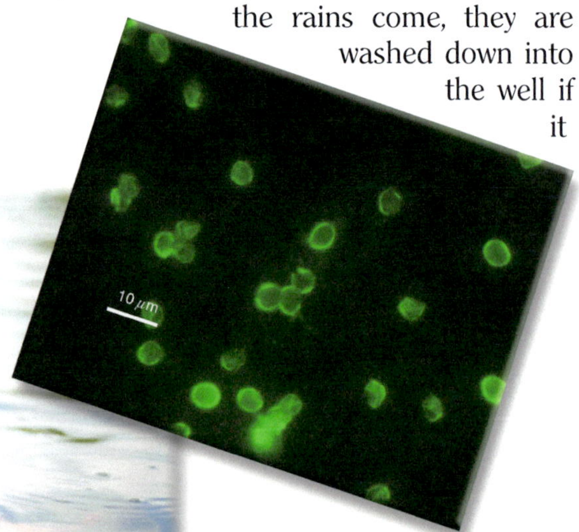

Cryptosporidium parvum are a microscopic parasite carried by impure water, often found in public swimming areas that lack filtration.

is near by. You can see some of the things found in bad water in the illustration on the next page.

It is best not to drink iced water when the body is heated, or during meals. If it is necessary to drink very cold water, the bad effects may be avoided by sipping it very slowly.

Tea and Coffee–Many people drink tea or coffee at their meals, and some persons think that these drinks are useful foods; but they really have little or no value as foods. Both tea and coffee contain a poison which, when separated in a pure form, is so deadly that a very small quantity is enough to kill a cat or a dog. This poison often does much harm to those who drink tea or coffee very strong for any great length of time.

Alcohol (al´-kuh-hall)–All of you know something about alcohol. Perhaps you have seen it burn in a lamp. It will burn without a lamp, if we light it. It is so clear and colorless that it looks like water. The Indians call it "fire-water." Alcohol differs very much from foods. It is not produced from plants, as fruits and grains are; neither is it supplied by Nature ready for our use, as are air and water.

Fermentation–When a baker makes bread he puts some yeast in the dough to make it "rise," so the bread will be light. The yeast destroys some of the sugar and starch in the flour and changes it into alcohol and a gas. The gas bubbles up through the dough, and this is what makes the bread light. This is called fermentation (fur-men-tay´-shun). The little alcohol which is formed in the bread does no harm, because it is all driven off by the heat when the bread is baked.

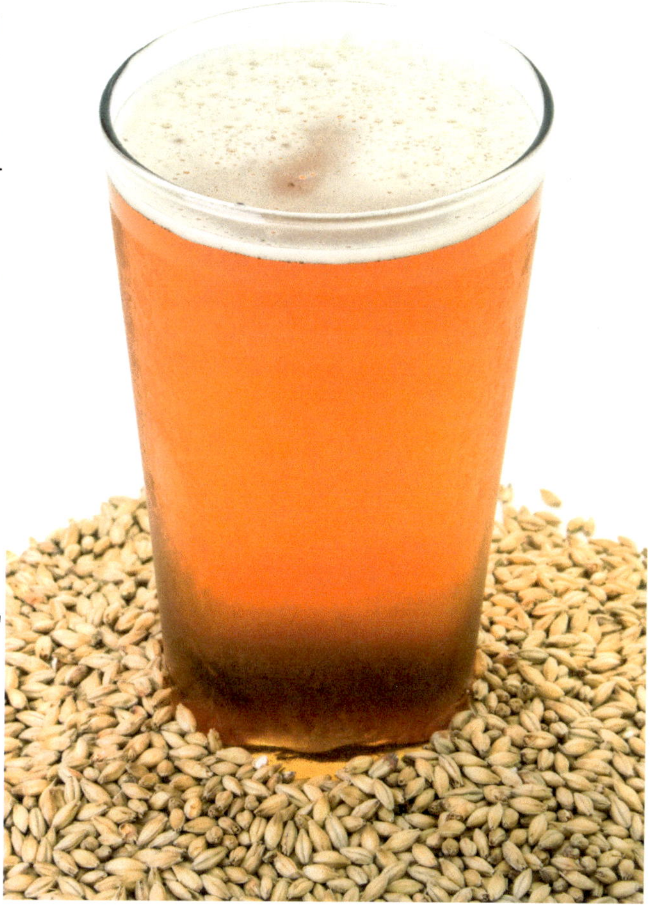

Any moist substance or liquid which contains sugar will ferment if yeast is added to it, or if it is kept in a warm place. You know that canned fruit sometimes spoils. This is because it ferments. Fermentation is a sort of decay. When the juice of grapes, apples, or other fruit is allowed to stand in a warm place it "works," or ferments, and thus produces alcohol. Wine is fermented grape-juice; hard cider is fermented apple-juice.

Beer, ale, and similar drinks are made from grains. The grain is first moistened and allowed to sprout. In sprouting, the starch of the grain is changed to sugar. The grain is next dried and ground, and is then boiled with water. The water dissolves the sugar. The sweet liquid thus obtained is separated from the grain, and yeast is added to it. This causes it to ferment, which changes the sugar to alcohol. Thus we see that the grain does not contain alcohol in the first place, but that it is produced by fermentation.

All fermented liquids contain more or less alcohol, mixed with water and a good many other things.

Distillation

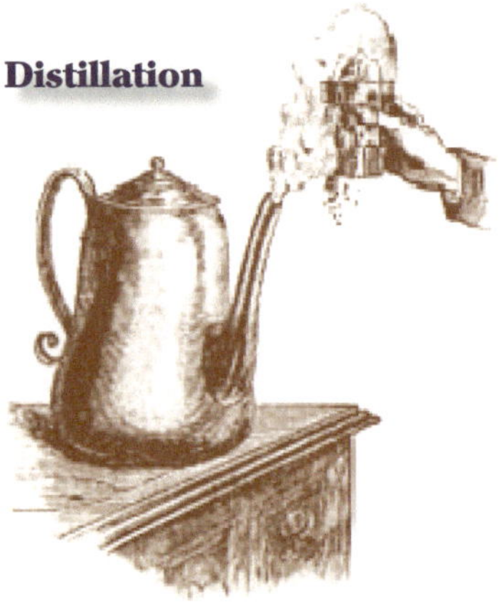

Rum, brandy, gin, whiskey, and pure alcohol are made by separating the alcohol from the other substances. This is done by means of a still, and is called distillation.

Alcohol Kills Animals and Plants–Strong alcohol has a deadly effect upon all living things. Once a man gave a dog a few tablespoonfuls of alcohol, and in a little while the dog was dead. If you should pour alcohol upon a plant it would die very soon.

A man once made a cruel experiment. He put some minnows into a jar of water and then poured in a few teaspoonfuls of alcohol. The minnows tried very hard to get out, but they could not, and in a little while they were all dead, poisoned by the alcohol. A Frenchman once gave alcohol to some pigs with their food. They soon became sick and died.

An Experiment
PLEASE DO THIS WITH ADULT ASSISTANCE ONLY!

Supplies:
1 Teapot filled with water
1 Herbal tea bag
1 Stove
1 Drinking Glass filled with water and a few ice cubes

Instructions:
Put the tea bag in the teapot with water. Get the water in the teapot to a boil on the stove with steam coming out at the nozzle. Hold up to the nozzle a common drinking-glass filled with iced water, first taking care to wipe the outside of the glass perfectly dry.

What Happens?
Little drops of water will soon gather upon the side of the glass. If you touch these to the tongue you will observe that they taste of the tea. It is because a little of the tea has escaped with the steam and condensed upon the glass. This is distillation.

This is how a still separates alcohol. If the teapot had contained wine, or beer, or hard cider, the distilled water would have contained alcohol instead of tea. By distilling the liquid several times the alcohol may be obtained almost pure.

Alcohol Not a Food–There are some people who imagine that alcohol is good for food because it is made from fruits and grains which are good for food. This is a serious mistake. A person can live on the fruits or grains from which alcohol is made, but no one would attempt to live upon alcohol. If he did, he would soon starve to death. In fact, people have often died in consequence of trying to use whiskey in place of food.

We should remember, also, that people do not take alcohol as a food, but for certain effects which it produces, which are not those of a food, but of a poison.

Many people who would not drink strong or distilled liquors, think that they will suffer no harm if they use only wine, beer, or cider. This is a great mistake. These liquids contain alcohol, as do all fermented drinks. A person will become drunk or intoxicated by drinking wine, beer, or cider–only a larger quantity is required to produce the same effect as rum or whiskey.

Another very serious thing to be thought of is that if a person forms the habit of drinking wine, cider, or other fermented drinks, they become so fond of the effect they produce that they soon want some stronger drink, and thus they are led to use whiskey or other strong liquors. On this account it is not safe to use any kind of alcoholic drinks, either fermented or distilled. The only safe plan is to avoid the use of every sort of stimulating or intoxicating drinks.

It has been found by observation that those persons who use intoxicating drinks are not so healthy as those who do not use them, and, as a rule, they do not live so long.

This is found to be true not only of those who use whiskey and other strong liquors, but also of those who use fermented drinks, as wine and beer. Beer drinkers are much more likely to suffer from disease than those who are strictly temperate. It is often noticed by physicians that when a beer-drinker becomes sick or meets with an accident, he does not recover so readily as one who uses no kind of alcoholic drinks.

Alcoholic drinks not only make people unhealthy and shorten their lives, but they are also the cause of much poverty and crime and an untold amount of misery.

POINTS TO REMEMBER

1. Water is the only thing that will satisfy thirst.

2. In going through our bodies, water washes out many impurities. We also need water to soften our food.

3. The purest water is the best. Impure water causes sickness.

4. Good water has no color, taste, or odor.

5. Tea and coffee are not good drinks. They are very injurious to children, and often do older persons much harm.

6. Alcohol is made by fermentation.

7. Pure alcohol and strong liquors are made by distillation.

8. Alcohol is not a food, it is a poison. It kills plants and animals, and is very injurious to human beings.

9. Even the moderate use of alcoholic drinks produces disease and shortens life.

HOW WE DIGEST

Did you ever see a Venus flytrap? This curious plant grows in North Carolina. It is called a flytrap because it has on each of its leaves something like a steel-trap, by means of which it catches flies. You can see one of these traps in the picture. When a fly touches the leaf, the trap shuts up at once, and the poor fly is caught and cannot get away. The harder it tries to escape, the more tightly the trap closes upon it, until after a time it is crushed to death.

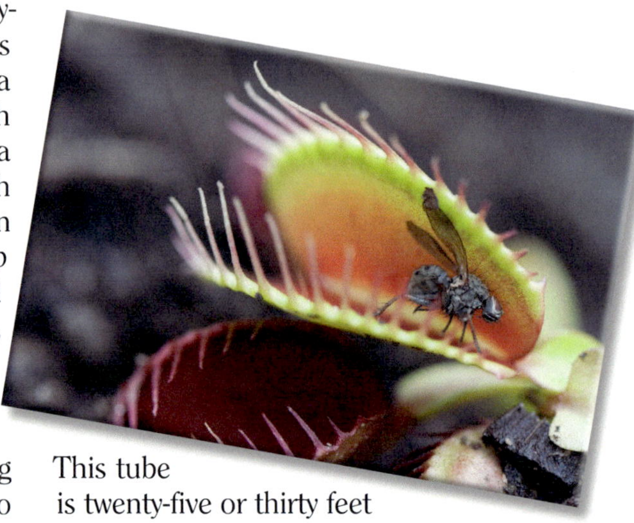

But we have yet to learn the most curious thing about this strange plant, which seems to act so much like an animal. If we open the leaf after a few days, it will be found that the fly has almost entirely disappeared. The fly has not escaped, but it has been dissolved by a fluid formed inside of the trap, and the plant has absorbed a portion of the fly. In fact, it has really eaten it. The process by which food is dissolved and changed so that it can be absorbed and may nourish the body, is called digestion (dy-jes´-shun).

The Venus flytrap has a very simple way of digesting its food. Its remarkable little trap serves it as a mouth to catch and hold its food, and as a stomach to digest it. The arrangement by which our food is digested is much less simple than this. Let us study the different parts by which this wonderful work is done.

The Digestive Tube–The most important part of the work of digesting our food is done in a long tube within the body, called the digestive tube or canal. This tube is twenty-five or thirty feet long in a full-grown man; but it is so coiled up and folded away that it occupies but little space. It begins at the mouth, and ends at the lower part of the trunk. The greater part of it is coiled up in the abdomen.

The Mouth–The space between the upper and the lower jaw is called the mouth. The lips form the front part and the cheeks the sides. At the back part are three openings. One, the upper, leads into the nose. There are two lower openings. One of these leads into the stomach, and the other leads to the lungs. The back part of the mouth joins the two tubes which lead from the mouth to the lungs and the stomach, and is called the throat. The mouth contains the tongue and the teeth.

The Teeth–The first teeth, those which come when we are small children, are called temporary or milk teeth. We lose these teeth as the jaws get larger and the second or permanent teeth take their place. There are twenty teeth in

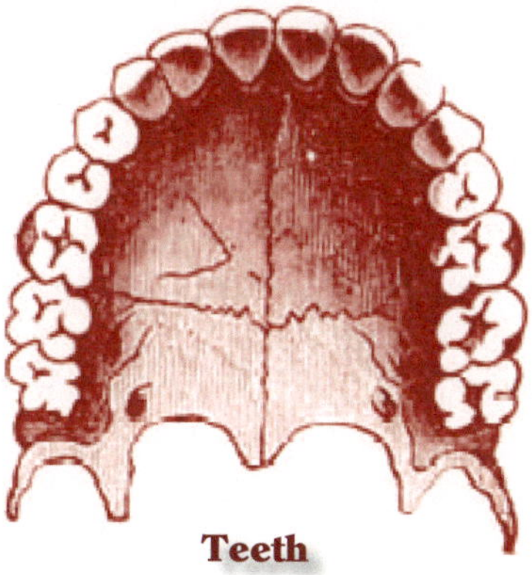

Teeth

the first set, and thirty-two in the second. Very old persons sometimes have a third set of teeth.

The Salivary (sal´-uh-var-ee) Glands–There are three pairs of salivary glands. They form a fluid called the saliva (sal-eye´-va). It is this fluid which moistens the mouth at all times. When we eat or taste something which we like, the salivary glands make so much saliva that we sometimes say the mouth waters. One pair of the salivary glands is at the back part of the lower jaw, in front of the ears. The other two pairs of glands are placed at the under side of the mouth. The saliva produced by the salivary glands is sent into the mouth through little tubes called ducts.

The Gullet–At the back part of the throat begins a narrow tube, which passes down to the stomach. This tube is about nine inches long. It is called the gullet, food-pipe, or esophagus (e-sof´-uh-gus).

The Stomach–At the lower end of the esophagus the digestive tube becomes enlarged, and has a shape somewhat like a pear. This is the stomach. In a full-grown person the stomach is sufficiently large to hold about three pints. At each end of the stomach is a narrow opening so arranged that it can be opened or tightly closed,

Gastric Gland

as may be necessary. The upper opening allows the food to pass into the stomach, the lower one allows it to pass out into the intestines (in-tes´-tins). This opening is called the pylorus (py-lo´-rus), or gate-keeper, because it closes so as to keep the food in the stomach until it is ready to pass out.

In the membrane which lines the stomach there

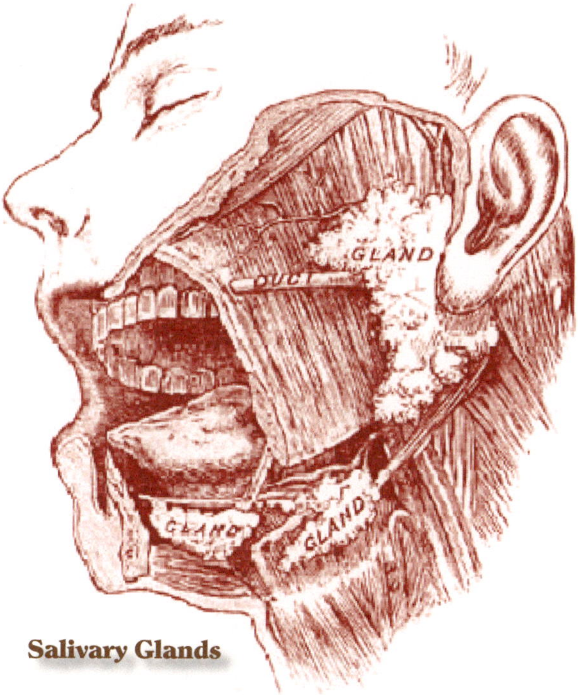

Salivary Glands

are many little pocket-like glands, in which a fluid called the gastric juice is formed. This fluid is one of the most important of all the fluids formed in the digestive canal.

The Intestine–At the lower end of the stomach the digestive canal becomes narrow again. This narrow portion, called the intestine, is about twenty-five feet long in a grown person. The last few feet of the intestine is larger than the rest, and is called the colon. This long tube is coiled up and snugly packed away in the cavity of the abdomen. In the membrane lining the intestines are to be found little glands, which make a fluid called intestinal juice.

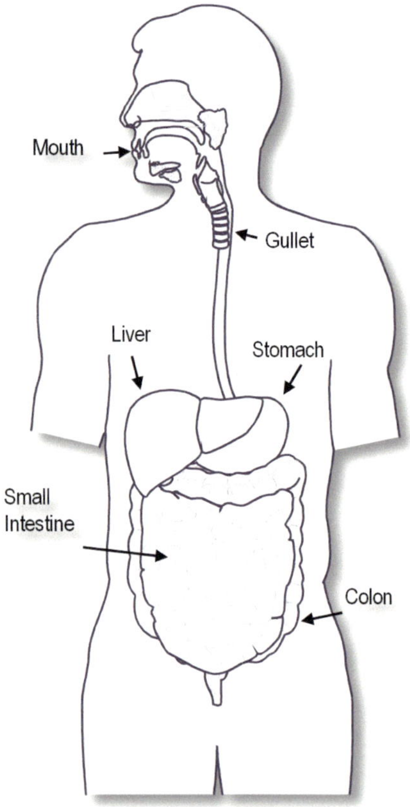

Digestive Tube

The Liver–Close up under the ribs, on the right side of the body, is a large chocolate-colored organ, called the liver. The liver is about half as large as the head, and is shaped so as to fit snugly into its corner of the abdomen. The chief business of the liver is to make a fluid called bile, which is very necessary for the digestion of our food.

The bile is a bitter fluid of a golden-brown color. It is carried to the intestine by means of a little tube or duct, which enters the small intestine a few inches below the stomach. When the bile is made faster than it is needed for immediate use, it is stored up in a little pear-shaped sac called the gall-bladder, which hangs from the under side of the liver.

The liver is a very wonderful organ, and does many useful things besides making bile. It aids in various ways in digesting the food, and helps to keep the blood pure by removing from it harmful substances which are formed within the body.

The Pancreas (pan´-kree-us)–The pancreas is another large and very important gland which is found close to the stomach, lying just behind it in the abdominal cavity. The pancreas forms a fluid called the pancreatic juice, which enters the small intestine at nearly the same place as the bile.

The Spleen–Close to the pancreas, at the left side of the body, is a dark, roundish organ about the size of the fist, called the spleen. It is not known that the spleen has much to do in the work of digestion, but it is so closely connected with the digestive organs that we need to know about it. The spleen works to destroy old red

Digestive System

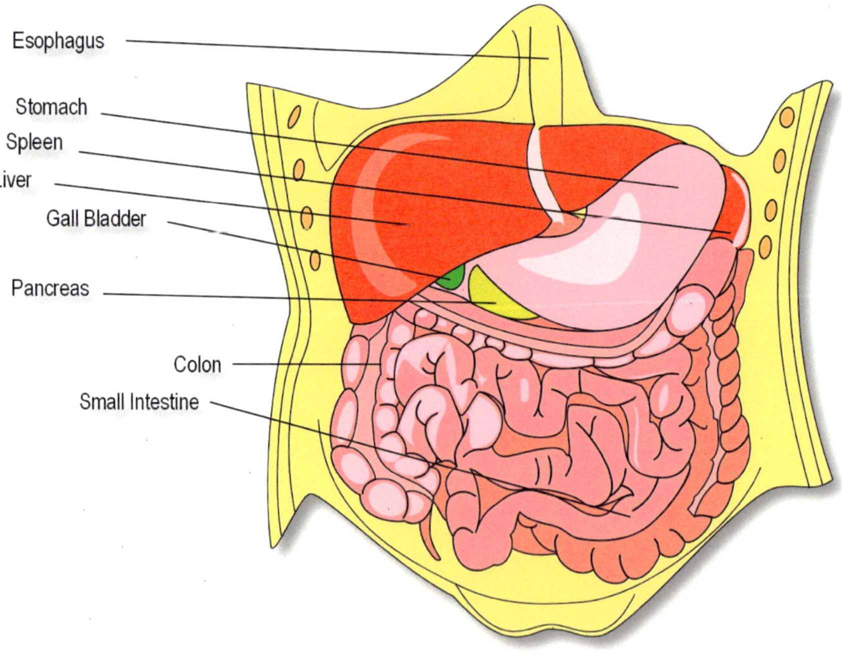

blood cells and stores platelets (plate´-lets) used for clotting blood when blood vessels break.

Please note that there are five important organs of digestion. The mouth, the stomach, the intestines, the pancreas, and the liver.

Also observe that there are five digestive fluids, saliva, gastric juice, bile, pancreatic juice, and intestinal juice.

POINTS TO REMEMBER

1. The process of dissolving and changing the food so that it may be absorbed and may nourish the body is digestion.

2. The work of digestion is chiefly done in the digestive tube or canal, which is about thirty feet in length.

3. The mouth contains the teeth, and has three pairs of salivary glands connected with it, which make saliva.

4. The gullet leads from the mouth to the stomach.

5. The stomach is pear-shaped, and holds about three pints.

6. It has an upper and a lower opening, each of which is guarded by a muscle, which keeps its contents from escaping.

7. The lower opening of the stomach is called the pylorus.

8. The stomach forms the gastric juice.

9. The intestines are about twenty-five feet long. They form the intestinal juice.

10. The liver lies under the ribs of the right side. It is about half as large as the head. It makes bile.

11. When not needed for immediate use, the bile is stored up in a sac called the gall-bladder.

12. The pancreas is a gland which lies just back of the stomach. It makes pancreatic juice.

13. The spleen is found near the pancreas.

14. There are five important digestive organs–the mouth, the stomach, the intestines, the liver, and the pancreas.

15. There are five digestive fluids–saliva, gastric juice, intestinal juice, bile, and pancreatic juice.

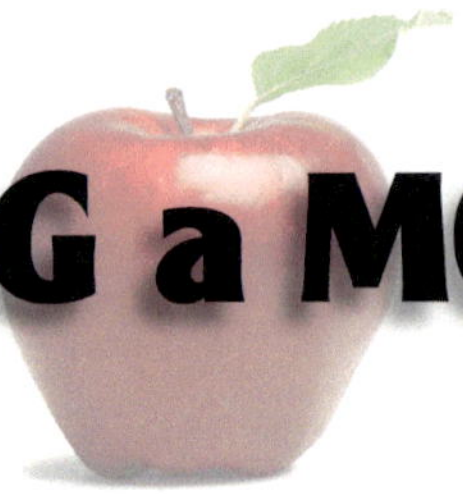

DIGESTING a MOUTHFUL

Let us suppose that we have eaten a mouthful of bread, and can watch it as it goes through all the different processes of digestion.

Mastication (mass-tuh-kay´-shun)–First, we chew or masticate the food with the teeth. We use the tongue to move the food from one side of the mouth to the other, and to keep the food between the teeth.

Mouth Digestion–While the bread is being chewed, the saliva is mixed with it and acts upon it. The saliva moistens and softens the food so that it can be easily swallowed and readily acted upon by the other digestive fluids. You have noticed that if you chew a bit of hard bread a few minutes it becomes sweet. This is because the saliva changes some of the starch of the food into sugar.

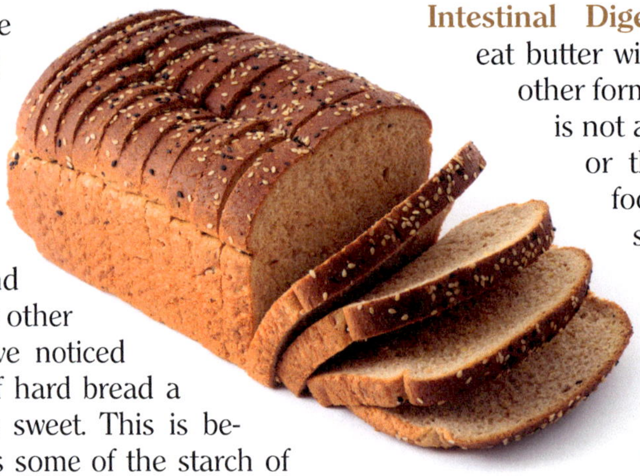

After we have chewed the food, we swallow it, and it passes down through the esophagus into the stomach.

Stomach Digestion–As soon as the morsel of food enters the stomach, the gastric fluid begins to flow out of the little glands in which it is formed. This mingles with the food and digests another portion which the saliva has not acted upon. While this is being done, the stomach keeps working the food much as a baker kneads dough. This is done to mix the gastric fluid with the food.

After an hour or two the stomach squeezes the food so hard that a little of it, which has been digested by the gastric fluid and the saliva, escapes through the lower opening, the pylorus, of which we have already learned. As the action of the stomach continues, more of the digested food escapes, until all that has been properly acted upon has passed out.

Intestinal Digestion–We sometimes eat butter with bread, or take some other form of fat in our food. This is not acted upon by the saliva or the gastric fluid. When food passes out of the stomach into the small intestine, a large quantity of bile is at once poured upon it. This bile has been made beforehand by the liver and stored up in the gall bladder. The bile helps to digest fats, which the saliva and the gastric fluid cannot digest.

The pancreatic fluid does the same kind of work that is done by the saliva, the gastric fluid, and the bile. It also finishes up the work done by these fluids. It is one of the most important of all the digestive fluids.

The intestinal fluid digests nearly all the different elements of the food, so that it is well fitted to complete the wonderful process by which the food is made ready to enter the blood and to nourish the body.

While the food is being acted upon by the bile, the pancreatic fluid, and intestinal fluid, it is gradually moved along the intestines. After all those portions of food which can be digested have been softened and dissolved, they are ready to be taken into the blood and distributed through the body.

Absorption–If you put a dry sponge into water, it very soon becomes wet by soaking up the water. Indeed, if you only touch a corner of the sponge to the water, the whole sponge will soon become wet. We say that the sponge absorbs the water. It is in a somewhat similar way that the food is taken up or absorbed by the walls of the stomach and intestines. When the food is absorbed, the greater part of it is taken into the blood vessels, of which we shall learn in a future lesson.

Liver Digestion–After the food has been absorbed, the most of it is carried to the liver, where the process of digestion is completed. The liver also acts like an inspector to examine the digested food and remove hurtful substances which may be taken with it, such as alcohol, mustard, pepper, and other irritating things.

The Thoracic (tho-ras´-ik) Duct–A portion of the food, especially the digested fats, is absorbed by a portion of the lymphatic vessels called lacteals (lak´-tee-als), which empty into a small vessel called the thoracic duct. This duct passes upward in front of the spine and empties into a vein near the heart.

POINTS TO REMEMBER

How a mouthful of food is digested:

1. It is first masticated–that is, it is chewed and moistened with saliva.

2. Then it is swallowed, passing through the esophagus to the stomach.

3. There it is acted upon, and a part of it digested by the gastric fluid.

4. It is then passed into the small intestine, where it is acted upon by the bile, the pancreatic fluid, and the intestinal fluid.

5. The digested food is then absorbed by the walls of the stomach and intestines.

6. The greater portion of the food is next passed through the liver, where hurtful substances are removed.

7. A smaller portion is carried through the thoracic duct and emptied into a vein near the heart.

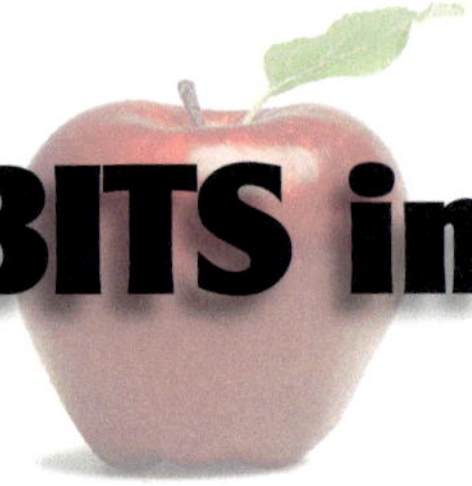

BAD HABITS in EATING

Eating too Fast–A most common fault is eating too fast. When the food is chewed too rapidly, and swallowed too quickly, it is not properly divided and softened. Such food cannot be easily acted upon by the various digestive juices.

Eating Too Much–A person who eats food too rapidly is also very likely to injure himself by eating too much. The digestive organs are able to do well only a certain amount of work. When too much food is eaten, none of it is digested as well as it should be. Food which is not well digested will not nourish the body.

Eating Too Often–Many children make themselves sick by eating too often. It is very harmful to take lunches or to eat at other than the proper meal times. The stomach needs time to rest, just as our legs and arms and the other parts of the body do. For the same reason, it is well for us to avoid eating late at night. The stomach needs to sleep with the rest of the body. If one goes to bed with the stomach full of food, the stomach cannot rest, and the work of digestion will go on so slowly that the sleep will likely be disturbed. Such sleep is not refreshing.

If we wish to keep our digestive organs in good order, we must take care to eat at regular hours. We ought not to eat when we are very tired. The stomach cannot digest well when we are very much fatigued.

Sweet Foods–We ought not to eat too much sugar or sweet foods, as they are likely to sour or ferment in the stomach, and so make us sick. Candies often contain a great many things which are not good for us, and which may make us sick. The colors used in candies are sometimes poisonous. The flavors used in them are also sometimes very harmful.

Fatty Foods Hurtful–Too much butter, fat meats, and other greasy foods are hurtful. Cream is the most digestible form of fat, because it readily dissolves in the fluids of the stomach, and mixes with the other foods without preventing their digestion. Melted fats are especially harmful. Cheese, fried foods, and rich pastry are very poor foods, and likely to cause sickness.

Eating Too Many Kinds of Foods–Children should avoid eating freely of flesh meats. They ought also to avoid eating all highly seasoned dishes, and taking too many kinds of food at a meal. A simple diet is much the more healthful. Milk and grain foods, as oatmeal, cracked wheat, graham bread, with such delicious fruits as apples, pears, and grapes, are much the best food for children.

Avoid Use of Cold Foods–We ought not to take very cold foods or liquids with our meals. Cold foods, ice-water, and other iced drinks make the stomach so cold that it cannot digest the food. For this reason it is very harmful to drink iced water or iced tea, or to eat ice-cream at meals. These things are injurious to us at any time, but they do the greatest amount of harm when taken with the food.

Things Sometimes Eaten Which are Not Foods–Things which are not foods are often used as foods, such as mustard, pepper, and the various kinds of seasonings. Soda, baking soda, and baking powders also belong to this class. All of these substances are more or less harmful, particularly mustard, pepper, and hot sauces.

Common Salt–The only apparent exception to the general rule that all condiments and other substances which are not foods are harmful is in the case of common salt. This is very commonly used among civilized nations, although there are many primitive tribes that never taste it. It is quite certain that much more salt is used than is needed. When too much salt is added to the food, the action of the digestive fluids is greatly hindered. Salt meats, and other foods which have much salt added to them, are hard to digest because the salt hardens the fibres of the meat, so that they are not easily dissolved by the digestive fluids.

Care of the Teeth–The teeth are the first organs employed in the work of digestion. It is of great importance that they should be kept in health. Many persons neglect their teeth, and treat them so badly that they begin to decay at a very early age.

The mouth and teeth should be carefully cleansed immediately on rising in the morning, and after each meal. All particles of food should be removed from between the teeth by carefully rubbing both the inner and the outer surfaces of the teeth with a soft brush and toothpaste, and rinsing very thoroughly with water. Daily use of floss is necessary to clean spaces between the teeth and to protect the gums from disease. The teeth should not be used in breaking nuts or other hard substances. The teeth are brittle, and are often broken in this way. The use of candy and too much sweet food is also likely to injure the teeth.

Some people think that it is not necessary to take care of the first set of teeth. This is a great mistake. If the first set are lost or are unhealthy, the second set will not be as perfect as they should be. It is plain that we should not neglect our teeth at any time of life.

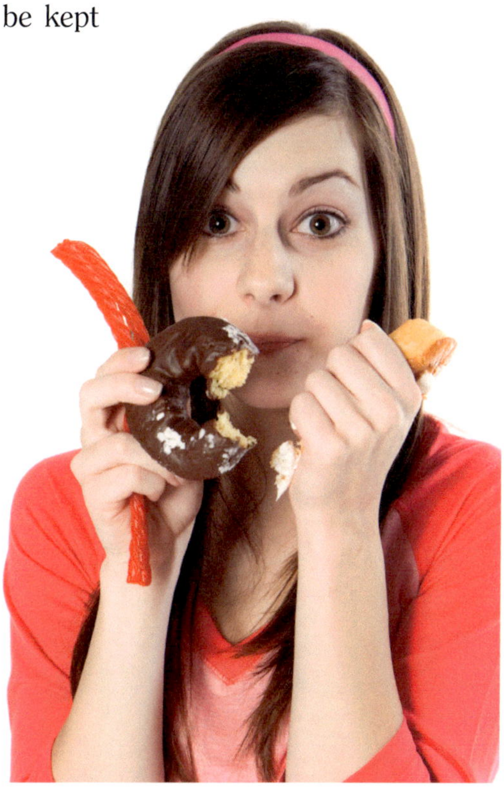

Tobacco–When a person first uses tobacco, it is apt to make him very sick at the stomach. After he has used tobacco a few times it does not make him sick, but it continues to do his stomach and other organs harm, and after a time may injure him very seriously. Smokers sometimes suffer from a horrible disease of the mouth or throat known as cancer.

Effects of Alcohol upon the Stomach–If you should put a little alcohol into your eye, the eye would become very red. When people take strong liquors into their stomachs, the delicate membrane lining the stomach becomes red in the same way. Perhaps you will ask how do we know that alcohol has such an effect upon the stomach. In 1822 there lived in Michigan a man named Alexis St. Martin. One day he was, by accident, shot in such a way that a large opening was made right through the skin and flesh and into the stomach. The good doctor who attended him took such excellent care of him that he got well. But when he recovered, the hole in his stomach remained, so that the doctor could look in and see just what was going on. St. Martin sometimes drank whiskey, and when he did, the doctor often looked into his stomach to see what the effect was, and he noticed that the inside of the stomach looked very red and inflamed.

POINTS TO REMEMBER

1. Causes of Indigestion.
   - ✓Eating too fast.
   - ✓Eating too much.
   - ✓Eating too frequently.
   - ✓Eating irregularly.
   - ✓Eating when tired.
   - ✓Eating too much of sweet foods.
   - ✓Eating too many kinds of food at a meal.
   - ✓Using iced foods or drinks.

2. Irritating substances and things which are not foods should not be eaten.

3. The teeth must be carefully used and kept clean.

4. Tobacco-using does the stomach harm, and sometimes causes cancer of the mouth.

5. Alcohol injures the gastric fluid, and causes disease of the stomach and the liver.

If St. Martin continued to drink whiskey for several days, the lining of the stomach looked very red and raw like a sore eye. A sore stomach cannot digest food well, and so the whole body becomes sick and weak. What would you think of a man who should keep his eyes always sore and inflamed and finally destroy his eyesight by putting pepper or alcohol or some other irritating substance into them every day? Is it not equally foolish and wicked to injure the stomach and destroy one's digestion by the use of alcoholic drinks? Alcohol, even when it is not very strong, not only hurts the lining of the stomach, but injures the gastric fluid, so that it cannot digest the food well.

Effects of Alcohol upon the Liver–The liver, as well as the stomach, is greatly damaged by the use of alcohol. You will recollect that nearly all the food digested and absorbed is filtered through the liver before it goes to the heart to be distributed to the rest of the body. In trying to save the rest of the body from the bad effects of alcohol, the liver is badly burned by the fiery liquid, and sometimes becomes so shriveled up that it can no longer produce bile and perform its other duties. Even beer, ale, and wine, which do not contain so much alcohol as do rum, gin, and whiskey, have enough of the poison in them to do the liver a great deal of harm, and to injure many other organs of the body as well.

A DROP of BLOOD

The Blood–Did you ever cut or prick your finger so as to make it bleed? Probably you have more than once met with an accident of this sort. All parts of the body contain blood. If the skin is broken in any place the blood flows out.

Do you know what a microscope is? It is an instrument which magnifies objects, or makes them look a great deal larger than they really are. Some microscopes are so powerful that they will make a little speck of dust look as large as a great rock.

The Blood Cells–If you should look at a tiny drop of blood through such a microscope, you would find it to be full of very small, round objects called blood cells.

You would notice also that these cells are of two kinds. Most of them are slightly reddish, and give to the blood its red color. A very few are white.

Use of the Cells–Do you wonder what these peculiar little cells do in the body? They are very necessary. We could not live a moment without them. We need to take into our bodies oxygen from the air. It is the business of the red cells to take up the oxygen in the lungs and carry it around through the body in a wonderful way, of which we shall learn more in a future lesson.

The white cells fight bacteria and viruses that enter the body . They are carried by the blood into all parts of the body and stop where they are needed to do any kind of work. They may be compared to the police who arrest criminals and remove them from the streets to keep the rest of us safe.

The cells float in a clear, almost colorless fluid which contains the digested food and other elements by which the body is nourished.

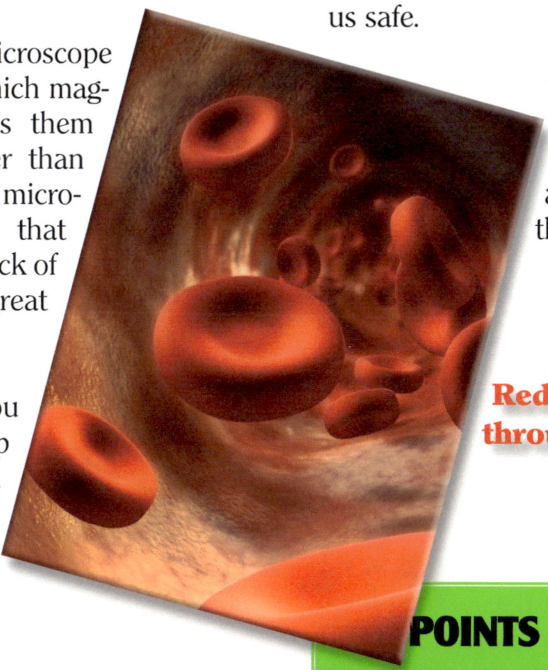

Red blood cells traveling through a blood vessel.

POINTS TO REMEMBER

1. The blood contains very mall objects called blood cells.

2. There are two kinds of cells, red and white.

3. The red cells carry oxygen.

4. The white cells repair parts that are worn.

5. The cells float in a clear, almost colorless fluid, which nourishes the body.

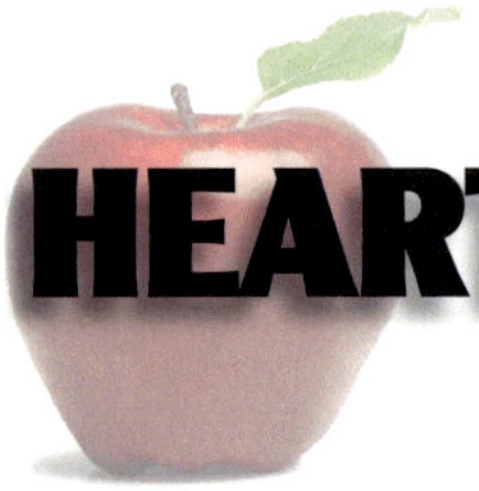

WHY the HEART BEATS

If you place your hand on the left side of your chest, you will feel something beating. If you cannot feel the beats easily, you may run up and down stairs two or three times, and then you can feel them very distinctly. Do you know the name of this curious machine inside the chest, that beats so steadily? You say at once that it is the heart.

The Heart–The heart may be called a live pump, which keeps pumping away during our whole lives. If it should stop, even for a minute or two, we would die. If you will place your hand over your heart and count the beats for exactly one minute, you will find that it beats about seventy-five or eighty times. When you are older, your heart will beat a little more slowly. If you count the beats while you are lying down, you will find that the heart beats more slowly than when you are sitting or standing. When we run or jump, the heart beats much harder and faster.

Why the Heart Beats–We have learned in preceding lessons that the digested food is taken into the blood. We have also learned that both water and oxygen are taken into the blood. Thus the blood contains all the materials that are needed by the various parts of the body to make good the wastes that are constantly taking place. But if the blood were all in one place it could do little good, as the new materials are needed in every part of the body. There has been provided a wonderful system of tubes running through every part of the body. By means of these tubes the blood is carried into every part where it is required. These tubes are connected with the heart. When the heart beats, it forces the blood through the tubes just as water is forced through a pipe by a pump or by a fire-engine.

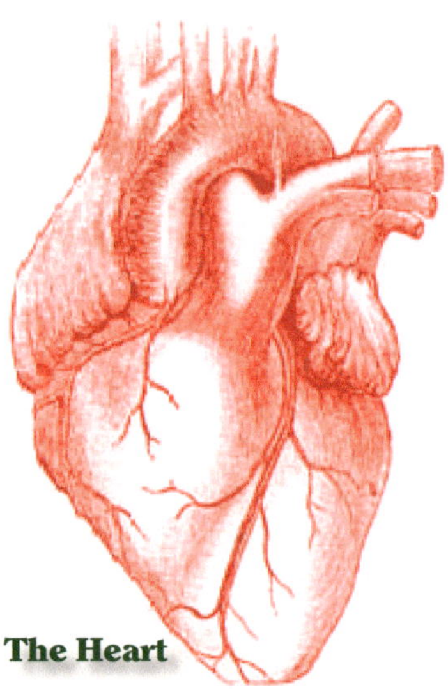

The Heart

The Heart Chambers–The heart has four chambers, two upper and two lower chambers. The blood is received into the upper chambers, and is then passed down into the lower cham-

The Inside of the Heart

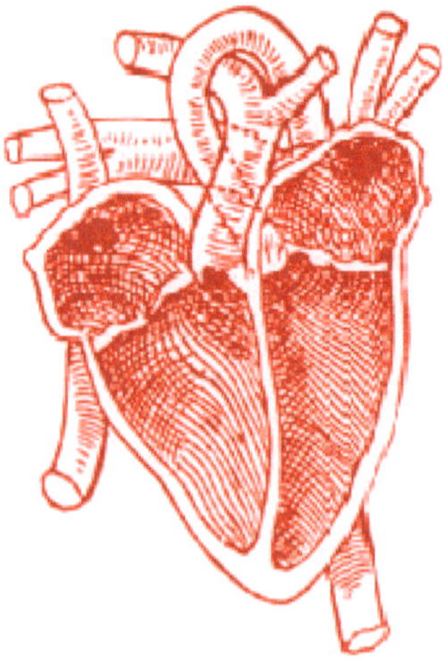

bers. From the lower chambers it is sent out to various parts of the body.

The Blood Vessels–The tubes through which the blood is carried are called blood-vessels. There are three kinds of blood-vessels. One set carry the blood away from the heart, and are called arteries (ar´-tuh-rees). Another set return the blood to the heart, and are called veins. The arteries and veins are connected at the ends farthest from the heart by many very small vessels. These minute, hairlike vessels are called capillaries (cap´-ul-la-rees).

The Arteries–An artery leads out from the lower chamber of each side of the heart. The one from the right side of the heart carries the blood only to the lungs. The one from the left side of the heart carries blood to every part of the body. It is the largest artery in the body, and is called the aorta. Soon after it leaves the heart the aorta begins to send out branches to various organs. These divide in the tissues again and again until they become so small that only one cell can pass through at a time.

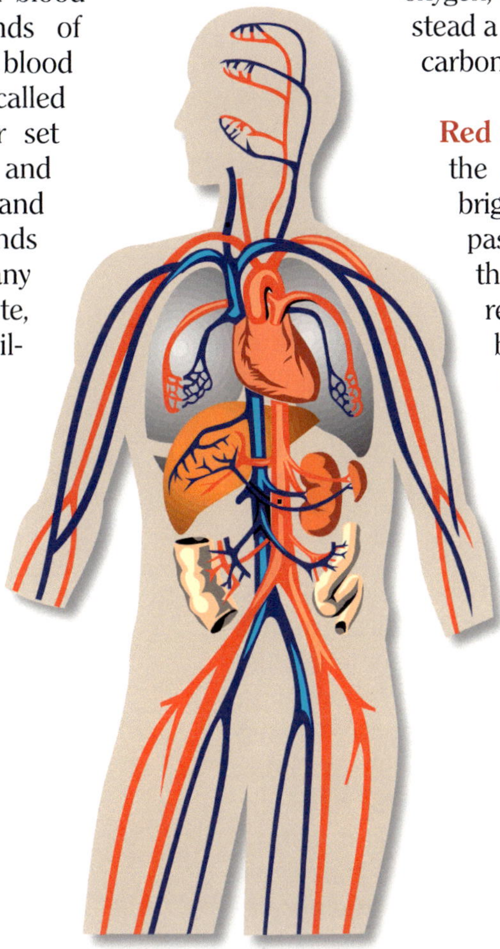

The Circulatory System

The Veins–These very small vessels now begin to unite and form larger ones, the veins. The small veins join to form larger ones, until finally all are gathered into two large veins which empty into the upper chamber of the right side of the heart. The veins which carry blood from the lungs to the heart empty into the upper chamber of the left side of the heart.

What is Done in the Blood Vessels–While the blood is passing through the small blood vessels in the various parts of the body, each part takes out just what it needs to build up its own tissues. At the same time, the tissues give in exchange their worn-out or waste matters. The red blood cells in the capillaries give up their oxygen, and the blood receives in its stead a poisonous substance called carbonic-acid gas.

Red and Blue Blood–While in the arteries the blood is of a bright red color; but while it is passing through the capillaries the color changes to a bluish red or purple color. The red blood is called arterial blood, because it is found in the arteries. The purple blood is called venous blood, because it is found in the veins. The loss of oxygen in the cells causes the change of color.

Change of Blood in the Lungs–Exactly the opposite change occurs in the blood when it passes through the lungs. The blood which has been gathered up from the various parts of the body is dark, impure blood. In the lungs this dark blood is spread out in very minute capillaries and exposed to the air. While passing through the capillaries of the lungs, the blood gives up some of its impurities in exchange for oxygen from the air. The red cells absorb the oxygen and the color of the blood changes from dark purple to bright red again. The purified blood is then carried back to the upper chamber of the left side of the heart through four large veins. The blood is now ready to begin another journey around the body.

The Pulse–If you place your finger on your wrist at just the right spot, you can feel a slight beating. This beating is called the pulse. It is caused by the movement of the blood in the artery of the wrist at each beat of the heart. The pulse can be felt at the neck and in other parts of the body where an artery comes near to the surface.

How Much Work the Heart Does–The heart is a small organ, only about as large as your fist, and yet it does an amount of work which is almost beyond belief. Each time it beats, it does as much work as your arm would do in lifting a large apple from the ground to your mouth. It beats when we are asleep as well as when we are awake. When we run we know by the way in which it beats that it is working very fast. Do you know how much a ton is? Well, in twenty-four hours the heart does as much work as a person would do in lifting stones enough to weigh more than one hundred and twenty tons.

The Lymphatic (lim–fat´-ik) System–The whole body is filled with small channels called lymphatics or lymph vessels which run together much like the meshes of a net. The lymphatic system is an important part of the body's defense against disease. As blood circulates through the body, fluid leaks into the body's organs supplying food to the body's many cells and absorbing waste back into the bloodstream. Lymphatics remove extra fluid from the body. They also produce the white blood cells, the cells that fight bacteria and viruses. In the center of the body the small lymphatics run into large ones, which empty into the veins near the heart.

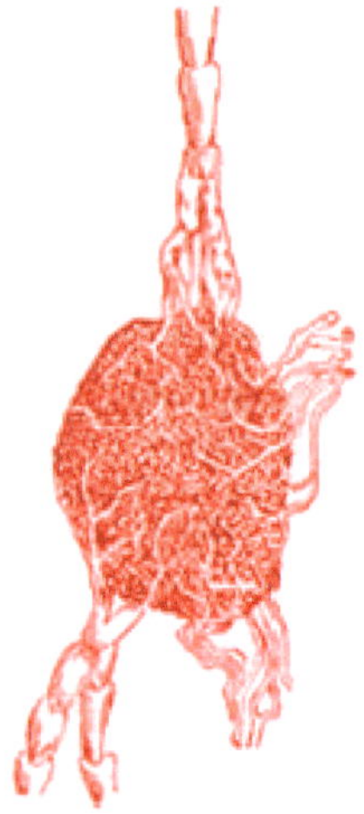

Lymph Node and Vessels

The Lymph–In the lymph channels the white cells float in a colorless fluid called lymph. The lymph is composed of the fluid portion of the blood which has soaked through the walls of the small vessels. The chief purpose of the lymphatics is to carry the lymph from the tissues back to the heart.

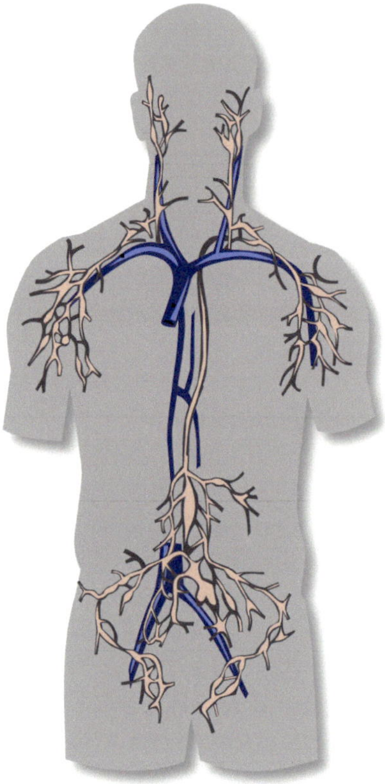

The Lymphatic System

Lymph Nodes–Here and there, scattered through the body, are oval structures into each of which many lymphatic vessels are found to run, as shown in the illustration. These are called lymph nodes. Lymph nodes are traps for particles that do not belong in the body, such as bacteria and viruses.

The heart and blood vessels are among the most wonderful structures in the body. It is no wonder, then, that alcohol, tobacco, and other narcotics and stimulants produce their most deadly effects upon these delicate organs. What these effects are we shall learn more fully in the next chapter.

POINTS TO REMEMBER

1. The heart beats to circulate the blood.

2. The heart has four chambers, two upper and two lower.

3. There are tubes called blood vessels which carry the blood to all parts of the body.

4. These tubes are connected with the heart.

5. The vessels which carry blood away from the heart are called arteries, and those which carry blood back to the heart are called veins.

6. The arteries and veins are connected by small tubes called capillaries.

7. The blood found in the arteries is red; that in the veins is dark blue or purple.

8. The color of the blood changes from red to blue in going through the capillaries. The change is due to the loss of oxygen.

9. In the circulation of the lungs, the blood in the arteries is blue, that in the veins, red.

10. The change from blue to red takes place while the blood is passing through the capillaries of the lungs. The change is due to the oxygen which the cells of the blood take up in the lungs.

11. The pulse is caused by the beating of the heart.

12. The heart does a great deal of work every day in forcing the blood into different parts of the body.

13. The lymphatic system helps protect the body against bacteria and viruses.

14. Lymph nodes are found throughout the body and act as traps for bacteria and viruses.

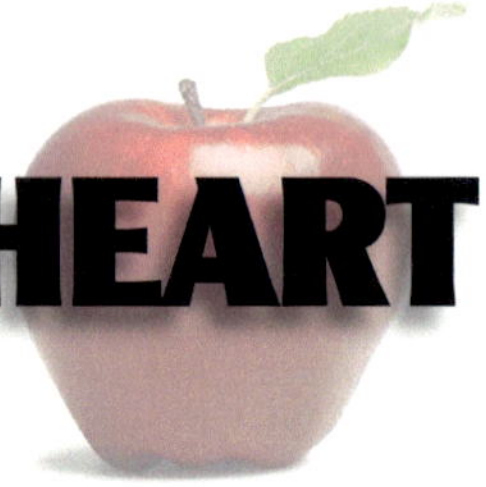

A HEALTHY HEART and BLOOD

The heart is one of the most important of all the organs of the body. If we take good care of it, it will do good service for us during a long life. Let us notice some ways in which the heart is likely to be injured.

Violent Exercise–Did you ever run so hard that you were out of breath? Do you know why you had to breathe so fast? It was because the violent exercise made your heart beat so rapidly that the blood could not get out of the lungs as fast as the heart forced it in. The lungs became so filled with blood that they could not do their work well. Sometimes, when a person runs very fast or takes any kind of violent exercise, the lungs become so filled with blood that a blood vessel is broken. The person may then bleed to death. It is very unwise to overtax the heart in any way, for it may be strained or otherwise injured, so that it can never again do its work properly.

Effects of Bad Air–Bad air is very harmful to the heart and to the blood also. We should always remember that the blood of the body while passing through the lungs is exposed to the air which we breathe. If the air is impure, the blood will be poisoned. Inside buildings with no fresh air and in other places where the air becomes foul, people often faint from the effects of the impure air upon the heart. It is important that the air of the rooms in which we live and sleep should be kept very pure by good ventilation.

Effects of Bad Food–The blood is made from what we eat, and if we eat impure and unwholesome food, the blood becomes impure. We ought to avoid the use of rich or highly-seasoned foods, candies, and all foods which are not nutritious. They not only injure the blood by making it impure, but they cause poor digestion.

Lack of Sleep–If we should take a drop of blood from the finger of a person who had not had as much sleep as he needed, and examine it with a microscope, we should find that there were too few of the little red blood cells. This is one reason why a person who has not had sufficient sleep looks pale.

Improper Clothing–We should be properly clothed, according to the weather. In cold weather we need very warm clothing. In warm weather we should wear lighter clothing. Our clothing should be so arranged that it will keep all parts of the body equally warm, and thus allow the blood to circulate properly. The feet are apt to be cold, being so far away from the heart, and we should take extra pains to keep them warm and dry.

Effects of Excessive Heat–In very hot weather, many persons are injured by exposing themselves to the sun too long at a time. Persons who drink alcoholic beverages are very often injured in this way, and sometimes die of sunstroke.

Effects of Anger–When a person gets very angry, the heart sometimes almost stops beating. Indeed, persons have died instantly in a fit of passion. So you see it is dangerous for a person to allow himself to become very angry.

Effects of Alcohol upon the Blood–If you should take a drop of blood upon your finger, and put it under the microscope, and then add a little alcohol to it, you would see that the cells would be quickly destroyed. In a few seconds they would be so shriveled up that no one could tell that they had ever been the beautiful little cells which are so necessary to health. When alcohol is taken as a drink, it does not destroy the cells so quickly, but it injures them so that they are not able to do their work of absorbing and carrying oxygen well. This is one reason why the faces of men who use alcoholic drinks often look so blue.

Alcohol Overworks the Heart–Dr. E. A.. Parkes, a very learned English physician, took the pains to observe carefully the effects of alcohol upon the heart of a soldier who was addicted to the use of liquor. He counted the beats of the soldier's pulse when he was sober; and then counted them again when he was using alcohol, and found that when the soldier took a pint of gin a day his heart was obliged to do one fourth more work than it ought to do.

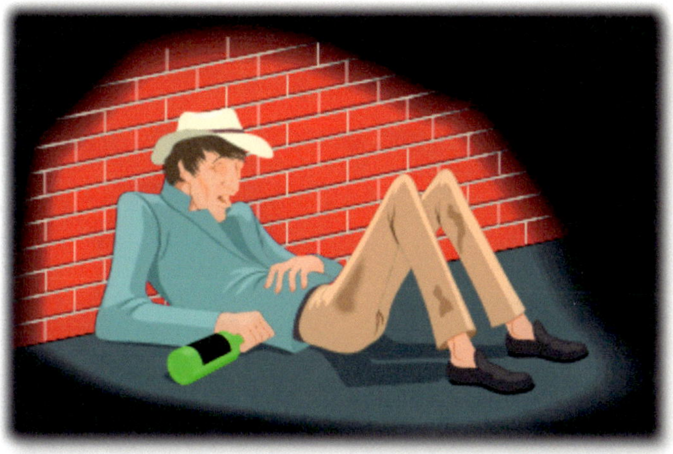

Effects of Alcohol upon the Blood Vessels–If you put your hands into warm water, they soon become red. This is because the blood vessels of the skin become enlarged by the heat, so that they hold more blood. Alcohol causes the blood to come to the surface in the same way. It is this that causes the flushed cheeks and the red eyes of the drunkard. Sometimes, after a man has been using alcohol a long time, the blood-vessels of his face remain enlarged all the time. This makes his nose grow too fast, and so in time it gets too large, and then he has a rum-blossom.

Effects of Tobacco on the Heart and the Blood–When a child first tries to use tobacco, it makes him feel very sick. If you should feel the pulse just then, you would find it very weak. This means that the heart is almost paralyzed by the powerful poison of the tobacco. Tobacco also injures the blood cells.

Effects of Caffeine-Tea, coffee and caffeinated drinks also do their share of mischief to the heart. Those who use them very strong often complain of palpitation (pal´-puh-ta-shun), or heavy and irregular beating of the heart.

Taking Cold–People often "catch cold" by allowing the circulation to become disturbed in some way, as by getting the feet wet, being chilled from not wearing sufficient clothing, sitting in a draught, and in other similar ways. This appears to lower the immune response of white cells that fight bacteria and viruses. It is very important for you to know that a cold is a serious thing, and should be carefully avoided. Protect yourself by dressing for cold weather, washing your hands before eating or after visiting places where there are ill persons, and practicing good eating habits.

Hemorrhage (hem'-or-ridge) or Loss of Blood–A severe loss of blood is likely to occur as the result of accidents or injuries of various sorts, and it is important to know what to do at once, as there may not be time to send for a doctor before it will be too late to save the injured person's life. Here are a few things to be remembered in all such cases:

If the blood from a cut or other wound flows in spurts, and is of a bright red color, it is from an artery. If it is dark-colored, and flows in a steady stream, it is from a vein.

How to Stop the Bleeding of Wounds–If the bleeding vessel is an artery, apply pressure on the side of the wound next to the heart. If the bleeding is from a vein, apply it on the opposite side. It is generally best to apply pressure directly over the wound or on both sides. The pressure can be made with the thumbs or with the whole hand. Grasp the part firmly and press very hard, or tie a handkerchief or towel around the wounded part and twist it very tight. If an arm or limb is the part injured, the person should be made to lie down, and the injured part should be held up. This is of itself an excellent means of stopping hemorrhage.

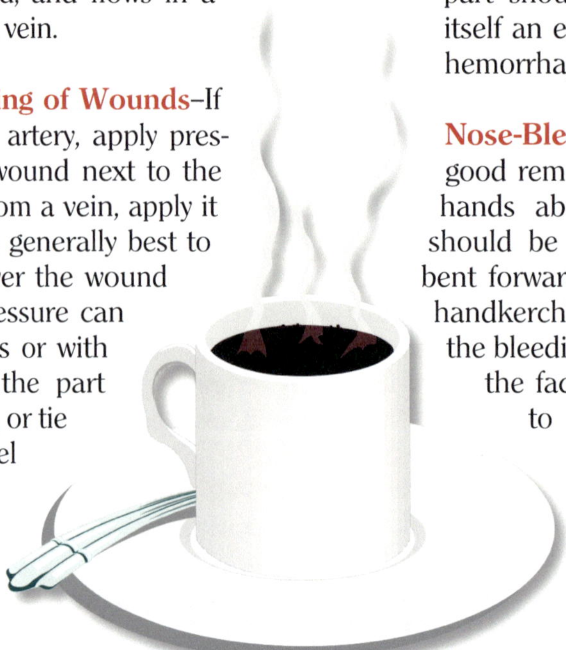

Nose-Bleed–For nose-bleed a very good remedy is holding one or both hands above the head. The head should be held up instead of being bent forward, and the corner of a dry handkerchief should be pressed into the bleeding nostril. It is well to bathe the face with very hot water, and to snuff hot water into the nostril if the bleeding is very severe. If the bleeding is very bad or is not readily stopped, a physician should be called.

POINTS TO REMEMBER

1. Violent exercise is likely to injure the heart.

2. Bad air makes the blood impure and disturbs the action of the heart.

3. Unwholesome food produces bad blood.

4. Too little sleep makes the blood poor.

5. Proper clothing is necessary to make the blood circulate equally in different parts of the body.

6. Violent anger may cause death by stopping the beating of the heart.

7. Alcohol injures the blood.

8. Alcohol overworks the heart.

9. Alcohol enlarges the blood vessels.

10. Tobacco injures the blood.

11. Tobacco weakens the heart and makes the pulse irregular.

12. The use of strong tea, coffee and other caffeinated drinks causes palpitation of the heart.

13. A cold can be caught by a disturbance of the circulation, making it harder for the body to fight bacteria and viruses. A cold should never be neglected.

14. When an artery is wounded, the blood is bright red and flows in spurts.

15. When a vein is wounded, the blood is purple and flows in a steady stream.

16. To stop bleeding from an artery, press on the side of the wound towards the heart, or on both sides of the wound.

17. When a vein is wounded, press on the side away from the heart.

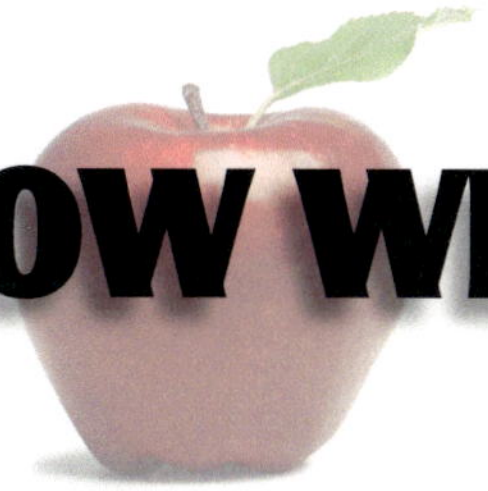

WHY and HOW WE BREATHE

In the experiment described on this page, what do you think is the reason that the candle will not burn when shut up in a bottle? A candle uses air when it burns. If shut up in a small, tight place, it soon uses up so much air that it can burn no longer. Try the experiment again, and when the candle begins to burn dimly, take it out quickly. We see that at once the light burns bright again.

Animals Die without Air–If you should shut up a mouse or any other small animal in a fruit jar, its life would go out just as the light of the candle went out. The little animal would die in a short time. A child shut up in a close place would die from the same cause in a very little time. In fact, many children are dying every day for want of a sufficient supply of pure air.

The Oxygen Experiment

PLEASE DO THIS WITH ADULT ASSISTANCE ONLY!

Supplies:
1 small candle
1 glass jar or bottle with a large mouth and lid
1 piece of wire about 1 foot long
1 match or lighter

Instructions:
Let us notice carefully what we are about to do and what happens. Fasten the candle to the end of the wire. Light it with a match or lighter, and let it down to the bottom of the jar. Now place the cover on the top of the jar and wait the results.

What Happens?
Soon the candle burns dimly and in a little time the light goes out altogether.

Oxygen–The reason why animals need air, and why the fire will not burn without it, is that the air contains oxygen, and it is the oxygen of the air which burns and produces heat. So it is the oxygen that burns in our bodies and keeps us warm.

When wood is burned in a fireplace, heat is produced; but some parts of the fuel are not made into heat. While the fire burns, smoke escapes through the chimney; but a part of the fuel remains in the fireplace in the form of ashes. Smoke and ashes are the waste parts of the fuel.

Poison in the Breath–The burning which takes place in our bodies produces something similar to the smoke and ashes produced by the fire in a fireplace. The smoke is called carbon dioxide gas, an invisible vapor, and escapes through the lungs. Do the experiment on this page to see how this works. The ashes are various waste and poisonous matters which are formed in all parts of the body. These waste matters are carried out of the body through the skin, the kidneys, the liver, and other organs.

Why We Breathe–By the experiment on page 41 we learn another reason why we breathe. We must breathe to get rid of the carbon dioxide gas, which is brought to the lungs by the blood to be exchanged for oxygen. There are two reasons then why we breathe: (a) to obtain oxygen; (b) to get rid of carbon dioxide gas.

The Lungs–Did you know we have an air-bag in our bodies. Our air-bag has to be emptied and filled often. We call this air-bag the lungs. We have learned before that the lungs are in the chest. Our lungs work like a pair of bellows. Let us now study our breathing-bellows and learn how they do their work.

The Windpipe and Air-tubes–A large tube called the windpipe or trachea (tray´-kee-uh) extends from the root of the tongue down the middle of the chest. The windpipe divides into two main branches, which subdivide again and again, until the finest branches are not larger than a sewing needle. The branches are called bronchial (bron´-key-ul) tubes. At the end of each tube is a cluster of small cavities called air-cells. The air-tubes and air-cells are well shown on the following page.

The Voice-box–If you will place the ends of your fingers upon your throat just above the breast-bone, you will feel the windpipe, and may notice the ridges upon it. These are rings of cartilage, a hard substance commonly called gristle. The purpose of these rings is to keep the windpipe open. Close under the chin you can find something which feels like a lump, and which moves up and down when you swallow.

This is a little box made of cartilage, called the voice-box (or larynx), because by means of this curious little apparatus we are able to talk and sing. Two little white bands are stretched across the inside of the voice-box. When we speak, these bands vibrate just as do the strings of the piano. These bands are called the vocal cords.

The Epiglottis (ep-uh-glot´-tis)–At the top of the voice-box is placed a curious trap-door which can be shut down so as to close the entrance to the air-passages of the lungs. This little door has a name rather hard to remember. It is called the epiglottis. The cover of the voice-box closes whenever we swallow anything. This keeps food or liquids from entering the air passages. If we eat or drink too fast the voice-box will not have time to close its little door and prevent our being choked. Persons have been choked to death by trying to swallow their food

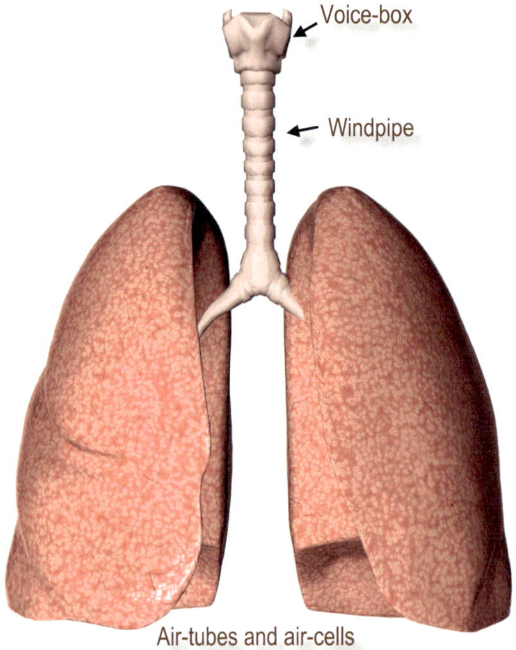

too fast. Do you not think this is a very wonderful door that can open and shut just when it should do so without our thinking anything about it?

The Nostrils and the Soft Palate–The air finds its way to the lungs through the mouth or through the two openings in the nose called the nostrils. From each nostril, three small passages lead backward through the nose. At the back part of the nasal cavity the passages of the two sides of the nose come together in an open space, just behind the soft curtain which hangs down at the back part of the mouth. This curtain is called the soft palate. Through the opening behind this curtain the air passes down into the voice-box and then into the lungs.

The Pleura (plur´-uh)–In the chest the air tubes and lung of each side are enclosed in a very thin covering, called the pleura. The cavity of the chest in which the lungs are suspended is also lined by the pleura. A limpid fluid flows from small openings in the pleura which keeps it moist, so that when the two surfaces rub together, as the lungs move, they do not become chafed and irritated.

Walls of the Chest–The ribs form a part of the framework of the chest. The ribs are elastic. The spaces between them are filled up with muscles, some of which draw the ribs together, while others draw them apart. Can you tell any reason why the walls of the chest are elastic? The lower wall or floor of the chest cavity is formed by a muscle called the diaphragm (dyuh´-fram), which divides the trunk into two cavities, the chest and the abdomen.

How We Use the Lungs–Now let us notice how we use the lungs and what takes place in them. When we use a pair of bellows, we take hold of the handles and draw them apart. The sides of the bellows are drawn apart so that there is more room between the sides. The air then rushes in to fill the space. When the bellows are full, we press the handles together and the air is forced out.

It is in just this way that we breathe. When we are about to take a long breath, the muscles pull upon the sides of the chest in such a way as to draw them apart. At the same time the diaphragm draws itself downward. By these means, the cavity of the chest is made larger and air rushes in through the nose or mouth to fill the space. When the muscles stop pulling, the walls of the chest fall back again to their usual position and the diaphragm rises. The cavity of the chest then becomes smaller and the air is forced out through the nose or mouth. This process is repeated every time we breathe.

We breathe once for each four heartbeats. Small children breathe more rapidly than grown persons. We usually breathe about eighteen or twenty times in a minute.

How Much the Lungs Hold–Every time we breathe, we take into our lungs about two thirds of a pint of air and breathe out the same quantity. Our lungs hold, however, very much more

The Carbon Dioxide Experiment

Supplies:
2 Drinking glasses, each filled with ½ cup of tap water
1 Drinking straw
1 lime

Instructions:
Have an adult cut the lime in half and squeeze the juice from each half into *one* of the drinking glasses. Now put one end of the straw into your mouth and place the other end in the pure water. Breathe through the tube a few times. Look at the water in the glass and see if a change has taken place. Now breathe through the lime-water in the other glass in the same way.

What Happens?
The pure water doesn't change at all. After breathing two or three times into the lime-water, you will notice that the water begins to look milky. In a short time it becomes almost as white as milk. This is because the lime-water catches the carbon dioxide gas which escapes from our lungs with each breath, while the pure water does not.

Bellows

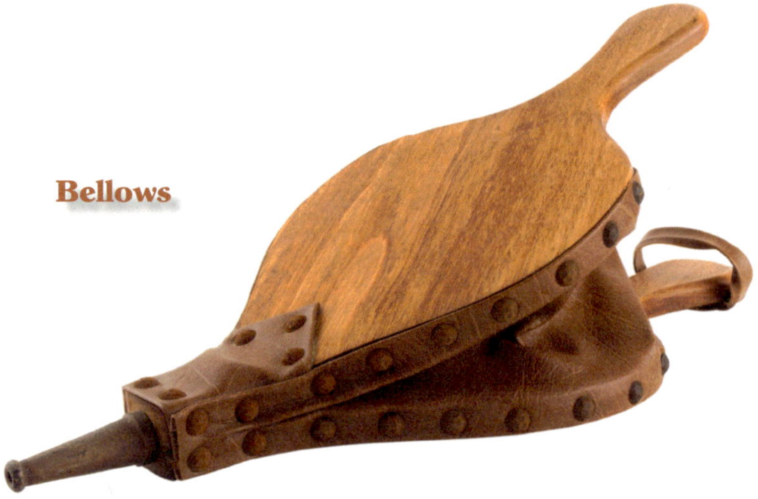

than this amount. A man, after he has taken a full breath, can breathe out a gallon of air, or more than ten times the usual amount. After he has breathed out all he can, there is still almost half a gallon of air in his lungs which he cannot breathe out. So you see the lungs hold almost a gallon and a half of air.

Do you think you can tell why God has given us so much more room in the lungs than we ordinarily use in breathing? If you will run up and down stairs three or four times you will see why we need this extra lung room. It is because when we exercise vigorously the heart works very much faster and beats harder, and we must breathe much faster and fuller to enable the lungs to purify the blood as fast as the heart pumps it into them.

The Two Breaths–We have learned that the air which we breathe out contains something which is not found in the air which we breathe in. This is carbon dioxide gas. How many of you remember how we found this out? We can also tell this in another way. If we put a candle down in a wide jar it will burn for some time. If we breathe into the jar first, however, the candle will go out as soon as we put it into the jar. This shows that the air which we breathe out contains something which will put a candle out. This is carbon dioxide gas, which is a poison and will destroy life.

Other Poisons–The air which we breathe out also contains other invisible poisons which are very much worse than the carbon dioxide gas. These poisons make the air of a crowded or unventilated room smell very unpleasant to one who has just come in from the fresh air. Such air is unfit to breathe.

The Lungs Purify the Blood–We have learned that the blood becomes dark in its journey through the body. This is because it loses its oxygen and receives carbon dioxide gas. While passing through the capillaries of the lungs, the blood gives out the carbon dioxide gas which it has gathered up in the tissues, and takes up a new supply of oxygen, which restores its scarlet hue.

How the Air is Purified–Perhaps it occurs to you that with so many people and animals breathing all the while, the air would after a time become so filled with carbon dioxide gas that it would be unfit to breathe. This is prevented by a wonderful arrangement of Nature. The carbon dioxide gas which is so poisonous to us is one of the most necessary foods for plants. Plants take in carbon dioxide gas through their leaves, and send the oxygen back into the air ready for us to use again.

We have already learned that the oxygen taken in by the lungs is carried to the various parts of the body by the little blood cells. The effect of strong alcoholic drinks is to injure these cells so that they cannot carry so much oxygen as they ought to do. For this reason, the blood of a drunkard is darker in color than that of a temperate person, and contains more carbon dioxide gas. The drunkard's lungs may supply all the air needed, but the blood has been so damaged that it cannot be used. Excessive smoking has a similar effect.

POINTS TO REMEMBER

1. Our bodies need air, just as a candle or a fire does.

2. A small animal shut up in a close jar soon dies for want of air. We need the oxygen which the air contains.

3. Oxygen causes a sort of burning in our bodies.

4. The burning in our bodies keeps us warm, and destroys some of the waste matters.

5. The breathing organs are the windpipe and bronchial tubes, the voice-box, the epiglottis, the nostrils, the soft palate, the lungs, the air-cells, the pleura, the diaphragm, and the chest walls.

6. When we breathe we use our lungs like a pair of bellows.

7. A man's lungs hold nearly one and a half gallons of air.

8. In ordinary breathing we use less than a pint of air, but when necessary we can use much more.

9. The air we breathe out contains carbon dioxide gas and another invisible poison.

10. A candle will not burn in air which has been breathed, and animals die when confined in such air.

11. The lungs purify the blood. While passing through the lungs, the color of the blood changes from purple to bright red.

12. Plants purify the air by removing the carbon dioxide gas.

13. Alcohol and tobacco injure the blood cells so that they cannot take up the oxygen from the air which the lungs receive.

KEEPING YOUR LUNGS HEALTHY

Pure Air Necessary–A person may go without eating for a month, or without drinking for several days, and still live; but a strong man will die in a few moments if deprived of air. It is very important that we breathe plenty of pure air. There are many ways in which the air becomes impure.

Bad Odors–Anything which rots or decays will in so doing produce an unpleasant odor. Bad odors produced in this way are very harmful and likely to make us sick. Garbage left to rot is dangerous to health, and gives rise to very serious disease in the big cities of many poor nations. We should always remember that bad odors caused by decaying substances are signs of danger to health and life, and that these substances should be removed from us, or we should get away from them, as soon as possible.

Germs–The chief reason why bad odors are dangerous is that they almost always have with them little living things called germs. Germs are so small that they cannot be seen by the naked eye: it takes a strong microscope to enable us to see them, but they are so powerful to do harm that if we receive them into our bodies they are likely to make us very sick, and they often cause death.

Contagious Diseases–You have heard about influenza (in´-flu-enza), pneumonia (new-mown´-ya), whooping cough and other contagious diseases. When a person is sick with one of these diseases, the air about him is poisoned with germs, which may give the same disease to other persons who inhale it. So when a person is sick from one of these diseases, it is very important that he should be put in a room by himself and shut away from every one but the doctor and the nurse. It is also necessary that all the clothing and bedding used by the sick person, and everything in the room, as well as the room itself, should be carefully cleansed and disinfected when the person has recovered, so as to wipe out every trace of the disease. The writer has known many cases in which persons who have been sick with some of these diseases were careless and gave the disease to others. Do you not think it very wrong for a person to give disease to another through carelessness.

Unhealthful vapors and odors of various sorts can arise from septic tanks and damp, close places under a poorly built house. Rooms which are shaded and shut up so closely that fresh air and sunshine seldom get into them should be avoided as dangerous to health.

Breath-Poisoned Air–The most dangerous of all the poisons to which we are exposed through the air are those of the breath, of which we learned in a preceding lesson. We need plenty of fresh air to take the place of the air which we poison by our breath. Every time we breathe, we spoil at least half a barrelful of air. We breathe twenty times a minute, and hence spoil ten barrels of air in one minute. How many barrels would this make in one hour? We need an equal quantity of pure air to take the place of the spoiled air, or not less than ten barrels every minute, or six hundred barrels every hour.

Ventilation–The only way to obtain the amount of fresh air needed, when we are shut up indoors, is to have some means provided by which the fresh air shall be brought in and the old and impure air carried out. Changing the air by such means is called ventilation. Every house, and especially every bedroom, should be well ventilated. Schools, churches, and other places where many people gather, need perfect ventilation. Ask your teacher to show you how the classroom is ventilated; and when you go home, talk to your parents about the ventilation of the house in which you live.

Many people ventilate their houses by opening the doors and windows. This is a very good way of ventilating a house in warm weather, but is a very poor way in cold weather, as it causes cold drafts, and makes the floor cold, so that it is difficult to keep the feet warm. It is much better to have the air warmed by a furnace or some similar means, before it enters the rooms. There ought also to be in each room a register to take the foul air out, so that it will not be necessary to open the windows. This register should be placed at the floor, because when the pure air enters the room warm, it first rises to the upper part of the room, and then as it cools and at the same time becomes impure, it settles to the floor, where it should be taken out by the register.

How to Breathe–We should always take pains to expand the lungs well in breathing, and to use the entire chest, both the upper and the lower part. Clothing should be worn in such a way that every portion of the chest can be expanded. For this reason it is very wrong to wear the clothing tight about the waist. Clothing so worn is likely to cause the lungs to become diseased.

Bad Habits–Students are very apt to make themselves flat-chested and round-shouldered by leaning over their desks while writing or studying. This is very harmful. We should always use great care to sit erect and to draw the shoulders well back. Then, if we take pains to fill the lungs well a great many times every day, we shall form the habit of expanding the lungs, and shall breathe deeper, even when we are not thinking about doing so.

Breathing through the Nose–In breathing, we should always take care to draw the air in

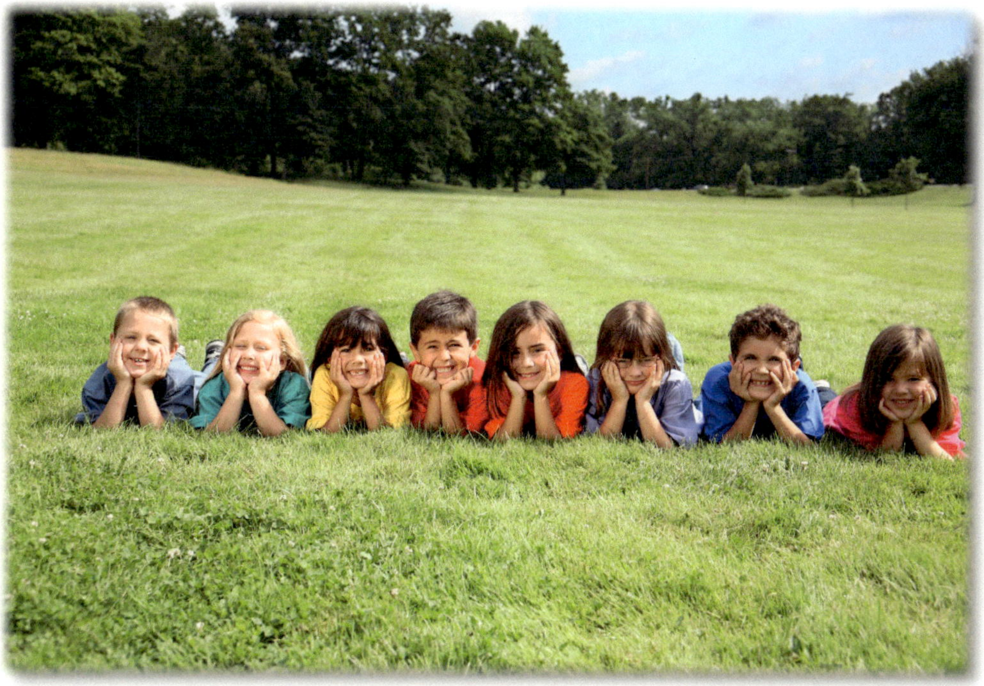

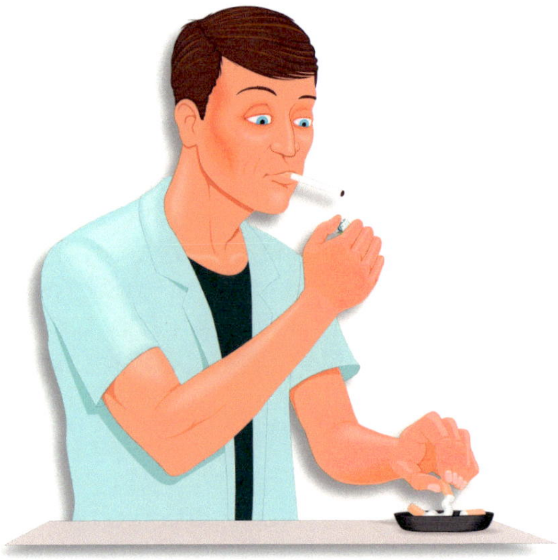

through the nose, and not through the mouth. The nose acts as a strainer, to remove particles of dust which might do harm if allowed to enter the lungs. It also warms and moistens the air in cold weather. The habit of breathing through the mouth often gives rise to serious disease of the throat and lungs.

Effects of Alcohol and Tobacco upon the Lungs–Both alcohol and tobacco produce disease of the breathing organs. Smoking injures the throat and sometimes causes loss of smell. Serious and even fatal diseases of the lungs are often caused by alcohol.

Many people suppose that the use of alcohol will save people from diseases. This is not true. A person may become a drunkard by the use of alcohol, and yet they is more likely to have disease than they would have been if they had been a total abstainer.

POINTS TO REMEMBER

1. Pure air is as necessary as food and drink.

2. Anything which is rotting or undergoing decay causes a bad odor, and thus makes the air impure.

3. Foul air contains germs which cause disease and often death.

4. Persons sick with contagious diseases should be carefully avoided. Such persons should be shut away from those who are well, and their rooms and clothing should be carefully cleansed and disinfected.

5. The breath poisons the air about us. Each breath spoils half a barrelful of air.

6. We should change the air in our houses, or ventilate them, so that we may always have pure air.

7. We should always keep the body erect, and expand the lungs well in breathing.

8. The clothing about the chest and waist should be loose, so that the lungs may have room to expand.

9. Always breathe through the nose.

10. Tobacco causes disease of the throat and nose.

11. Alcohol causes diseases and makes people more likely to become diseased.

The SKIN and WHAT IT DOES

The Skin–The skin is the covering of the body. It fits so exactly that it has the precise shape of the body, like a closely fitting garment. If you will take up a little fold of the skin you will see that it can be stretched like a piece of rubber. Like rubber, when it is released it quickly contracts and appears as before.

The Bark of Trees–Did you ever peel the bark off of a young tree? If so, you have noticed that there were really two barks, an outer bark, as thin as paper, through which you could almost see, and an inner and much thicker bark, which lay next to the wood of the tree. You can peel the outer bark off without doing the tree much harm. Indeed, if you will notice some of the fruit or shade trees in the yard, at home, you will see that the outer bark of the tree peels itself off, a little at a time, and that new bark grows in its place. If you tear off the inner bark, however, it will injure the tree. It will make it bleed, or cause the sap to run. The sap is the blood of the tree. The bark is the skin of the tree. When the bare place heals over, an ugly scar will be left.

The Epidermis (eh-puh´-dur-mus)–Our bodies, like trees, have more than one skin. We have three skins. When a person burns himself so as to make a blister, the outer skin, called the epidermis, is separated from the inner layers by a quantity of water or serum poured out from the blood. This causes the blister to rise above the surrounding skin. If you puncture the blister the water runs out. Now we may easily remove the epidermis and examine it. The epidermis, we shall find, looks very much like the skin which lines the inside of an egg shell, and it is almost as thin.

The epidermis is very thin in most parts of the body, but in some places, as the palms of the hands and the soles of the feet, it is quite thick. This is because these parts of the skin come in contact with objects in such a way as to be liable to injury if not thus protected. The epidermis has no blood vessels and very few nerves. With a fine needle and thread you can easily take a stitch in it without making it bleed or causing any pain.

The Pigment–The under side of the epidermis is colored by little particles of pigment or melanin (meh-luh´-nin). The color of this pigment differs in different races. In African persons, the color of the pigment is black. In some races the pigment is brown. In white persons there is very little pigment, and in some persons, called albinos, there is none at all.

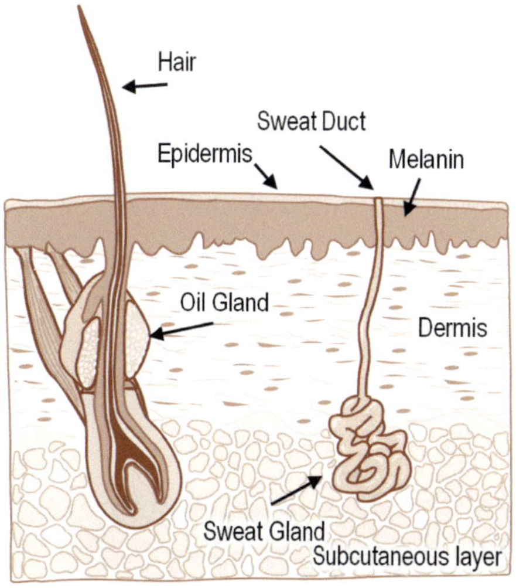

The Structure of the Skin

The Dermis (dur´-mus)–The inner skin, like the inner bark of a tree, is much thicker than the outer skin. It is much more important, and is called the dermis. It contains nerves and blood vessels.

The Subcutaneous (sub-kyoo-tay´-nee-us) Layer–The third layer of the skin below the dermis is the subcutaneous layer. It is made mostly of fat cells used to cushion the body against hard objects and to protect the body from cold. The hair begins its growth in this layer of the skin.

The Sweat Glands–If you look at the palm of the hand you will see many coarse lines, and by looking much closer you will see that the palm is completely covered with very fine ridges and furrows. Now, if you examine these ridges with a magnifying glass, you will find arranged along each ridge a number of little dark spots. Each of these points is the mouth of a very small tube. This is called a sweat duct. These ducts run down through both the outer and inner layers of the skin. At the under side of the true skin the end of the tube is rolled up in a coil, as you can see by looking at the illustration below The coiled parts of the tubes are called sweat glands, because they separate from the blood the fluid which we call sweat or perspiration.

The Oil Glands–There are other little glands in the skin which make oil. The oil is poured out upon the skin to keep it soft and smooth.

The Hair–There are some curious little pockets in the skin. Out of each of these pockets grows a hair. On some parts of the body the hairs are coarse and long; on other parts they are fine and short.

Many of the ducts leading from the oil glands open into the pockets or pouches from which the hairs grow. The oil makes the hair soft and glossy.

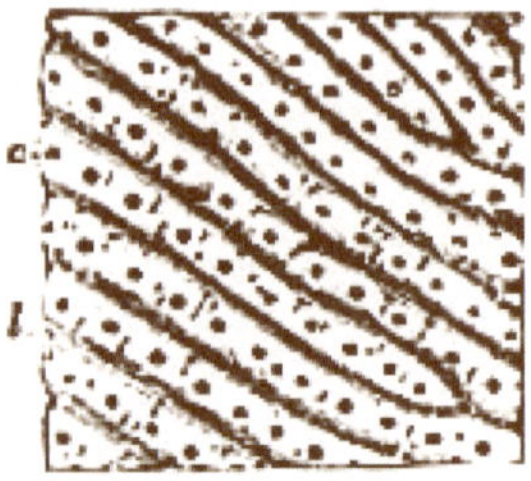

Skin of Palm of Hand Magnified

God has thus provided an excellent means for oiling the hair.

The hair is chiefly useful as a protection. It is also an ornament.

The Nails–The nails of the fingers and the toes grow out of little pockets in the skin just as the hairs do. Both the hair and the nails are really parts of the outer skin, which is curiously changed and hardened. The nails lie upon the surface of the dermis and grow from the under side as well as from the little fold of skin at the root of the nail. They are made to give firmness and protection to the ends of the fingers and toes. The nails of the fingers are also useful in picking up small objects and in many other ways.

Uses of the Skin–The skin is useful in several ways:

(1) *It Removes Waste*–The sweat glands and ducts are constantly at work removing from the blood particles which have been worn out and can be of no further use. If we get very warm, or if we run or work very hard, the skin becomes wet with sweat. In a little while, if we stop to rest, the sweat is all gone. What becomes of it? You say it dries up, which means that it has passed off into the air. Sweating is going on all the time, but we do not sweat so much when we are quiet and are not too warm, and so the sweat dries up as fast as it is produced, and we do not see it. Nearly a quart of sweat escapes from the skin daily.

(2) *Ventilation through the Skin*–We ventilate to a slight extent through the skin, releasing gases. There are some lower animals which breathe with their skins altogether. A frog can breathe with its skin so well that it can live for some time after its lungs have been removed. Ventilation is an important part of the work of the skin, and we should be careful, by keeping it clean and healthy, to give it a good chance to ventilate all that it can.

(3) *The Skin Absorbs*–The skin absorbs many substances which come in contact with it, and hence should be kept clean. If the foul substances which are removed in the sweat are allowed to remain upon the skin, they may be taken back into the system and thus do much harm.

(4) *The Skin has Feeling*–When anything touches the skin we know it by the feeling. We can tell a great many things about objects by feeling of them. If we happen to stick a pin into the skin we feel pain. We are also able to tell the difference between things which are hot and those which are cold. Thus the sense of feeling which the skin has is very useful to us.

(5) *The Skin Protects the Body*–The skin is a natural clothing which protects us much better than any other kind of clothing could. It is so soft and pliable that it cannot hurt the most delicate part which it covers, yet it is very strong and tough.

POINTS TO REMEMBER

1. The skin is the covering of the body. It has three layers, the outer, called the epidermis, the inner, called the dermis, and the third layer called the subcutaneous layer.

2. A substance called pigment, or melanin, is found between the epidermis and the dermis. This gives the skin its color.

3. The dermis has blood vessels and nerves, but the epidermis has no blood vessels and very few nerves.

4. In the dermis are glands which produce sweat, and others which make oil.

5. The subcutaneous layer contains fat cells.

6. The nails are really a part of the skin. They are firm and hard, and protect the ends of the fingers and the toes.

7. The hair grows from the subcutaneous layer. The hair is made soft and glossy by oil from the oil glands of the skin.

8. The skin is a very useful organ. It removes waste matters, it ventilates, it absorbs, it has feeling, and it protects the body.

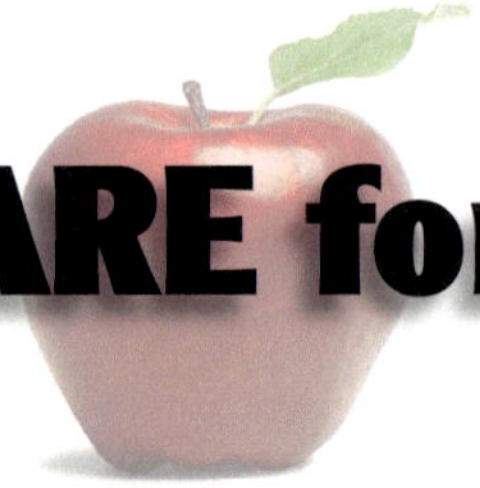

HOW to CARE for the SKIN

Uses of the Pores of the Skin–Many years ago, at a great celebration, a little boy was covered all over with varnish and gold leaf, so as to make him represent an angel. The little gilded boy looked very pretty for a short time, but soon he became very sick, and in a few hours he was dead. Can you guess what made him die? He died because the pores of his skin were stopped up, and the sweat glands could not carry off the poisonous matter from his body.

Cleanliness–Did you ever know of a boy who had his skin varnished? Not exactly, perhaps; but there are many boys who do not have their skins washed as often as they ought to be, and the sweat and oil and dead scales form a sort of varnish which stops up the little ducts and prevents the air from getting to the skin, almost as much as a coat of varnish would do.

The Sweat Glands–The sweat glands and ducts are like little sewers, made to carry away some of the impurities of the body. There are so many of them that, if they were all put together, they would make a tube two or three miles long. These little sewers drain off almost a quart of impurities in the form of sweat every day. So you see that it is very important for the skin to be kept clean and healthy.

Bathing–A bird takes a bath every day. Dogs and many other animals like to go into the water to bathe. You may have seen a great elephant take a bath by showering the water over himself with his trunk. To keep the skin healthy we should bathe frequently.

When we take a bath for cleanliness it is necessary to use a little soap, so as to remove the oil which is mixed up with the dry sweat, dead cells, and dirt which may have become attached to the skin.

It is not well to take hot baths very often, as they have a tendency to make the skin too sensitive. Bathing in cool water hardens the skin, and helps to strengthen the immune system.

The Clothing–The skin should be protected by proper clothing, but it is not well to wear more than is necessary..

The Proper Temperature of Rooms–It is also very unwise for a person to keep the rooms in which he lives too warm, and to stay too much indoors, as it weakens the immune system.

Care of the Hair and the Nails–The scalp should be kept clean by thorough and frequent washing and daily brushing. Hair oils are seldom needed. If the skin of the head is kept in a healthy condition, the hair requires no oil.

The habit of biting and picking the fingernails is a very unpleasant one, and keeps the nails in a broken and unhealthy condition. The nails should be carefully trimmed with nail clippers.

Effects of Narcotics and Stimulants upon the Skin–Alcohol, tobacco, opium, and all other narcotics and stimulants have a bad effect upon the skin. Alcohol often causes the skin to become red and blotched, and tobacco gives it a dingy and unhealthy appearance.

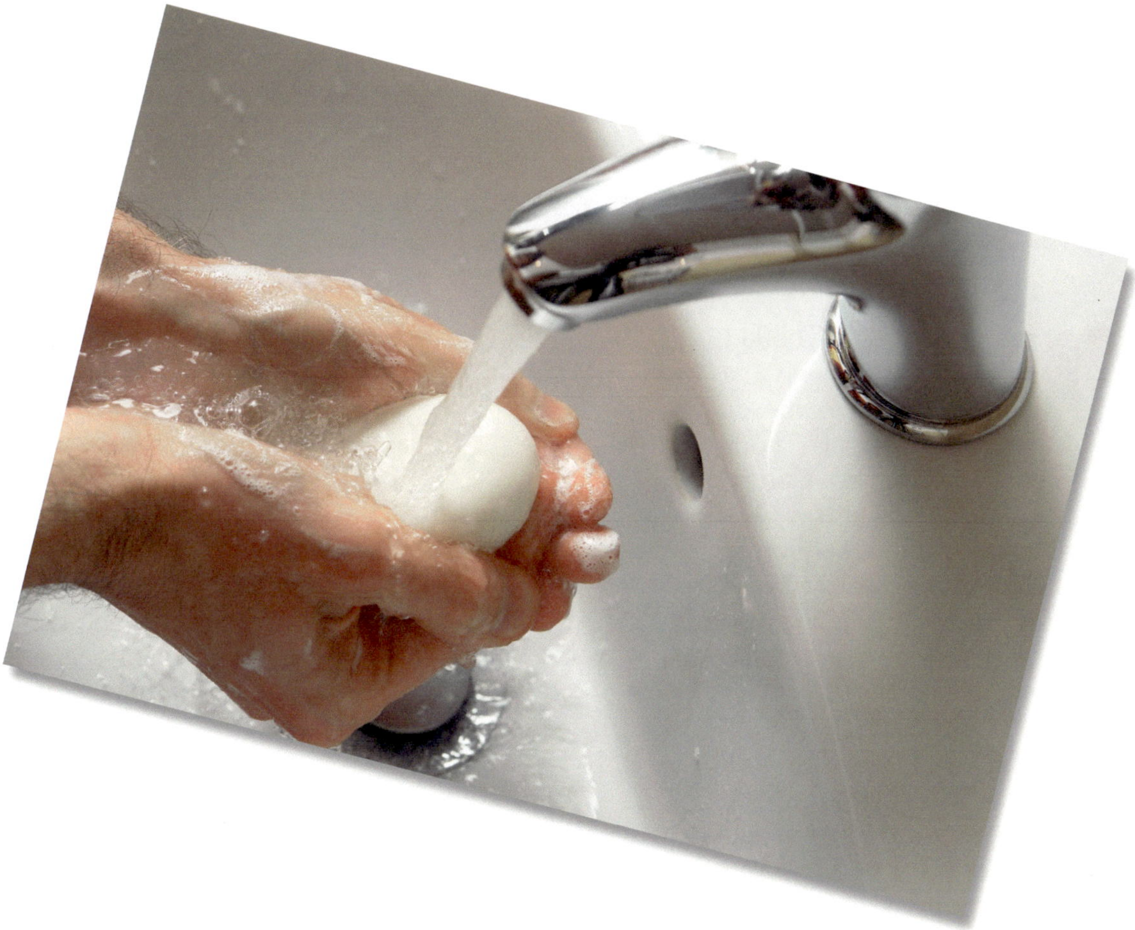

POINTS TO REMEMBER

1. If the pores of the skin are closed, a person will die.

2. We should bathe often enough to keep the skin clean.

3. We should not keep our rooms too warm, and should avoid wearing too much clothing.

4. Alcohol, tobacco, and other stimulants and narcotics injure the skin.

The KIDNEYS and THEIR WORK

The Kidneys–The kidneys are among the most important organs of the body. There are two kidneys in the cavity of the abdomen, near the backbone, up under the lower border of the ribs. Perhaps you have seen the kidneys of a sheep or a hog. If you have, you know very nearly how the kidneys of our own bodies appear.

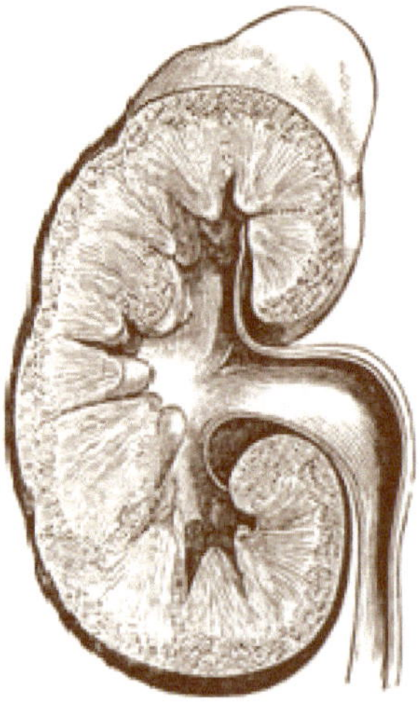

Kidney

The Work of the Kidneys–The work of the kidneys is to separate from the blood certain very poisonous substances, which would soon cause our death if they were not removed. It is very important to keep these useful organs in good health, because a person is certain to die very soon when the kidneys are in any way seriously injured.

How to Keep the Kidneys Healthy–One way of keeping the kidneys in good health is to drink plenty of pure water, and to avoid eating too much meat and rich food. Pepper, mustard, and other hot sauces are very harmful to the kidneys.

Importance of Keeping the Skin Clean–The work of the kidneys is very similar to that of the skin; and when the skin does not do its full duty, the kidneys have to do more than they should, and hence are likely to become diseased. For this reason, persons who allow their skins to become inactive by neglecting to bathe frequently are apt to have disease of the kidneys.

Effects of Alcohol and Tobacco upon the Kidneys–A piece of beef placed in alcohol soon becomes dry and hard, and shrivels up as though it had been burned. The effect upon the kidneys of drinking alcohol is almost the same. Beer and hard liquor also do the kidneys harm, sometimes producing incurable disease of these important organs.

POINTS TO REMEMBER

1. The kidneys somewhat resemble the skin in their structure and in their work.

2. The kidneys remove from the blood some poisonous substances.

3. To keep the kidneys healthy we should drink plenty of water, avoid irritating foods and drinks, and keep the skin in health by proper bathing.

4. The drinking of strong liquors often causes incurable disease of the kidneys.

OUR BONES and THEIR USES

The Bones–In an earlier chapter we learned something about the bones. This we must try to recall. You will remember that we called the bones the framework of the body, just as the timbers which are first put up in building a house are called its frame.

The Skeleton–All the bones together make up the skeleton. There are about two hundred bones in all. They are of many different shapes. They vary in size from the little bones of the ear, which are the smallest, to the upper bone of the leg or femur (fee´-mur), which is the largest in the body.

The skeleton is divided into four parts: the skull, the trunk, the arms, and the legs. We must learn something more about the bones of each part

The Skull–The skull is somewhat like a shell. It is made of a number of bones joined together in such a way as to leave a hollow place inside to hold the brain. The front part of the skull forms the framework of the face and the jaws. In each ear there are three curious little bones, which aid us in hearing.

The Trunk–The bones of the trunk are, the ribs, the sternum, the pelvis, and the spinal (spy´-nul) column. The bones of the trunk form a framework to support and protect the various organs within its cavities.

The Ribs–There are twelve ribs on each side. The ribs join the spinal column at the back.

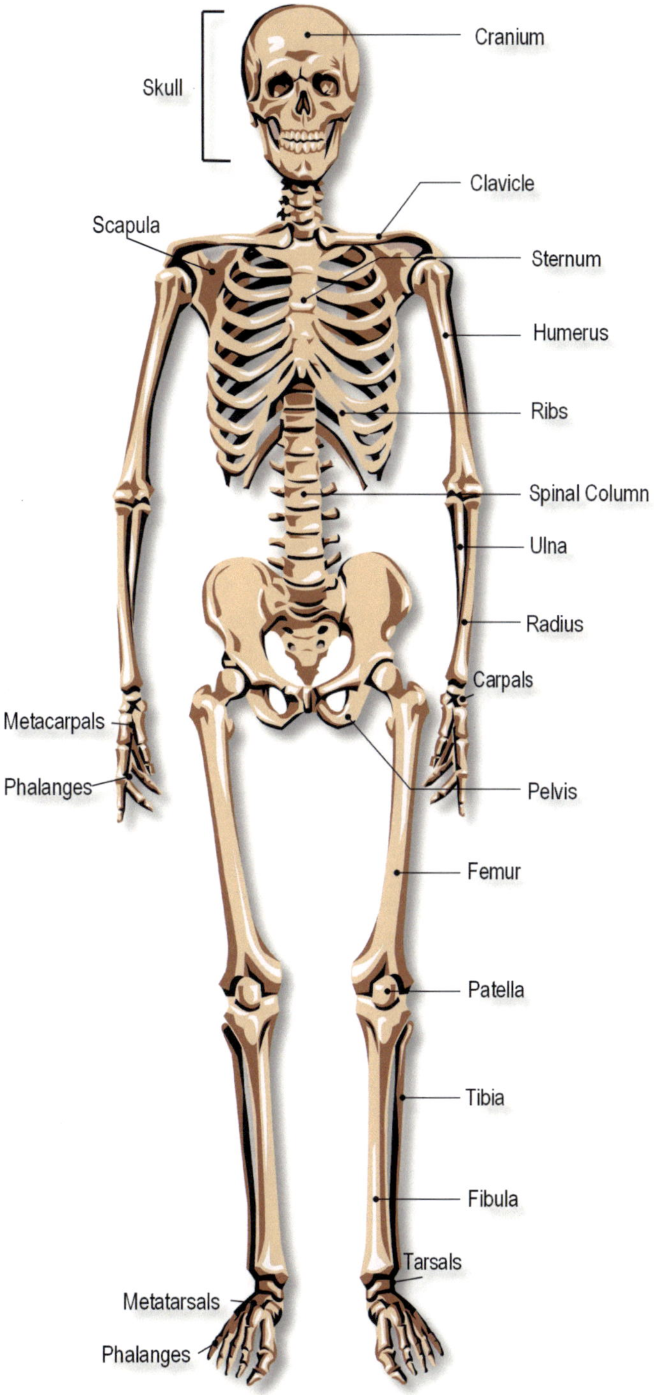

They are connected by cartilage to the sternum in front. They look somewhat like the hoops of a barrel. With the sternum and the spinal column they form a bony cage to contain and protect the heart and the lungs.

The Pelvis–The pelvis is at the lower part of the trunk. It is formed by three bones, closely joined together. The large bones at either side are called the hipbones. Each hipbone contains a deep round cavity in which the upper end of the femur rests.

The Spinal Column–The spinal column, or backbone, is made up of twenty-four small bones, joined together in such a way that the whole can be bent in various directions. The skull rests upon the upper end of the spinal column. The lower end of the spinal column forms a part of the pelvis.

The Spinal Canal–Each of the separate bones that make up the spinal column has an opening through it, and the bones are so arranged, one above another, that the openings make a sort of canal in the spinal column. By the connection of the spinal column to the head, this canal opens into the cavity of the skull. Through this canal there passes a peculiar substance called the spinal cord, of which we shall learn more at another time.

The Arms–Each of the arms has five bones, besides the small bones of the hand. They are the clavicle (klav´-i-kul), which connects the shoulder to the sternum, the scapula (skap´-u-luh), at the back of the shoulders, the humerus (hyu´-mer-us), between the shoulder and the elbow, and the two lower arm-bones called the radius (ray´-de-us) and ulna (ul´-nuh), between the elbow and the wrist. There are eight little bones in the wrist called the carpals (kar´-pulls), five in that part of the hand next to the wrist called metacarpals (meh-tuh-kar´-pulls), and fourteen in the fingers and thumb called phalanges (full-an´-jeez).

The Legs–The bones of the leg are the femur or upper leg-bone, the patella (puh-tel´-uh) or knee-cap, which covers the front of the knee. The two bones of the lower leg are called the tibia (tib´-ee-uh) and fibula (fib´-yoo-luh). In the foot there are the heel-bone and six other bones in the ankle called the tarsals (tar´-suls), five bones in that part of the foot next to the ankle called the metatarsals (meh-tuh-tar´suls), and fourteen bones in the toes called phalanges, like those of the fingers.

Use of the Bones–The skeleton is not only necessary as a framework for the body, but it is useful in other ways. Some of the bones, as the skull, protect delicate parts. The brain is so soft and delicate that it would be very unsafe without its solid bony covering. The spinal cord also needs the protection which it finds in the strong but flexible spinal column. The bones help to move our hands and arms, and assist us in walking.

The Joints–The places where two or more bones are fastened together are called joints. Some joints we can move very freely, as those of the shoulder and the hip. Others have no motion at all, as those of the bones of the skull.

Cartilage (cart´-uh-lij)–The ends of bones which come together to form a joint are covered with a smooth, tough substance, which protects the bone from wear. This is called cartilage.

The joint contains a fluid to oil it, so that the ends of the bones move upon each other very easily. If the joints were dry, every movement of the body would be very difficult and painful.

The bones are held together at the joints by means of strong bands called ligaments (lig´-a-ments).

How the Bones are Made–The bones are not so solid as they seem to be. The outside of most bones is much harder and firmer than the inside. Long bones, like those of the arms and the legs, are hollow. The hollow space is filled with marrow, in which are the blood vessels which nourish the bone. Red and white blood corpuscles (cells) are also produced in the marrow.

If one weighed a piece of bone, then burned it in the fire for several hours, and then weighed it again, they would find that it has lost about one third of its weight. They would also notice that it has become brittle, and that it seems like chalk.

Why the Bones are Brittle–The hard, brittle portion of a bone which is left after it has been burned contains a good deal of calcium (kahl´-see-um). It is this which makes the bones so hard and firm that they do not bend by the weight of the body. When we are young, the bones have less of this calcium, and so they bend easily, and readily get out of shape.

A person's height depends upon the length of their bones. The use of alcohol and tobacco by a growing child has a tendency to stunt the growth of the bones, so that they do not develop as they should.

POINTS TO REMEMBER

1. There are about two hundred bones in the body.

2. All together they are called the skeleton.

3. The skeleton is divided as follows:

   a. The Skull

   b. The Trunk
      - ✓ Ribs
      - ✓ Sternum
      - ✓ Pelvis
      - ✓ Spinal column

   c. The Arms
      - ✓ Clavicle
      - ✓ Scapula
      - ✓ Humerus
      - ✓ Radius and Ulna
      - ✓ Carpals
      - ✓ Metacarpals and Phalanges

   d. The Legs
      - ✓ Femur
      - ✓ Patella
      - ✓ Tibia and Fibula
      - ✓ Tarsals
      - ✓ Metatarsals and Phalanges

4. The bones are useful for support, protection, and motion.

5. The place where two bones join is called a joint.

6. The tough substance which covers the ends of many bones is called cartilage.

7. The joints are enabled to work easily by the aid of a fluid secreted for that purpose.

8. The ends of the bones are held together in a joint by means of ligaments.

9. Calcium gives bones their hardness.

10. The use of alcohol and tobacco may prevent proper development of the bones.

KEEPING YOUR BONES HEALTHY

Composition of the Bones–Our bones, like the rest of our bodies, are made of what we eat. If our food does not contain enough of the substances which are needed to make healthy bone, the bones will become unhealthy. They may be too soft and become bent or otherwise misshapen. This is one of the reasons why bread made from the whole grain is so much more healthful than that made from very fine white flour. In making fine white flour the miller takes out the very best part of the grain, just what is needed to make strong and healthy bones. Oatmeal is a very good food for making healthy bones.

Bones of Children–When a child is born, the bones are soft. They harden as the child grows older and becomes an adult.

Improper Positions–The bones are so soft and flexible when we are young that they are very easily bent out of shape if we allow ourselves to take improper positions in sitting, lying, or standing. This is the way in which flat and hollow chests, uneven shoulders, curved spines, and many other deformities are caused.

In sitting, standing, and walking, we should always take care to keep the shoulders well back and the chest well expanded, so that we may not grow misshapen and deformed. The illustrations on this page and the next show good and bad positions and also the effects of bad positions.

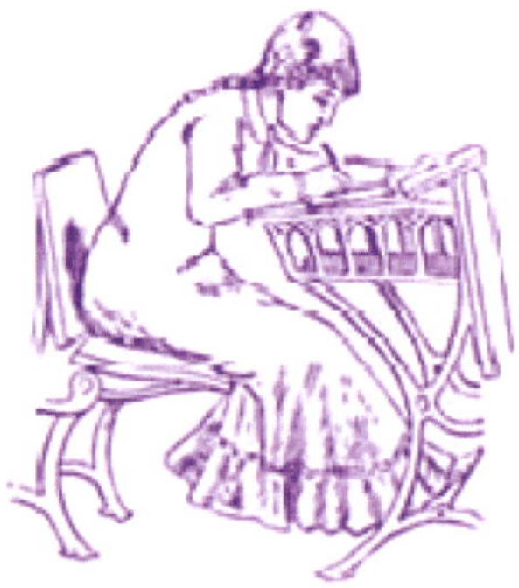

Improper Position

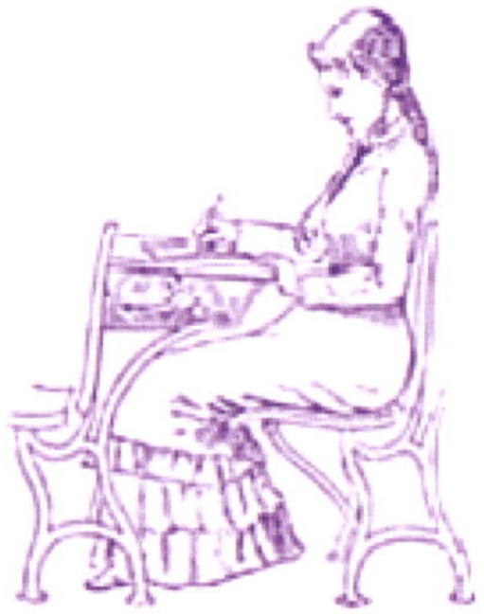

Proper Position

Seats and Desks–The seats and desks of school children should be of proper height. The seats should be low enough to allow the feet to rest easily upon the floor, but not too low. The desk should be of such a height that, in writing, one shoulder will not be raised above the other. If a young person bends the body forward, he will, after a time, become round-shouldered and his chest will become so flattened that the lungs cannot be well expanded.

Standing on one foot, sitting bent forward when reading or at work, sleeping with the head raised high upon a thick pillow or bolster, are ways in which young persons can grow out of shape.

The Clothing–Wearing the clothing tight about the waist often produces serious deformities of the bones of the trunk, and makes the chest so small that the lungs have not room to act properly. Tight or high-heeled shoes also often deform and injure the feet and make the gait stiff and awkward.

Broken Bones–By rough play or by accident the bones may be broken in two just as you might break a stick. If the broken parts are placed right, they will cement together making the bone strong again.

Sprains–In a similar manner the ligaments which hold the bones together, in a joint, are sometimes torn or over-stretched. Such an accident is called a sprain. A sprain is a very painful accident, and a joint injured in this way needs to rest quite a long time so that the torn ligaments may grow together.

Bones Out of Joint–Sometimes the ligaments are torn so badly that the ends of the bones are displaced, and then we say they are put out of joint. This is a very bad accident indeed, but it often happens to boys while wrestling or playing at other rough games.

Children sometimes have a trick of pulling the fingers to cause the knuckles to "crack." This is a very foolish and harmful practice. It weakens the joints and causes them to grow large and unsightly.

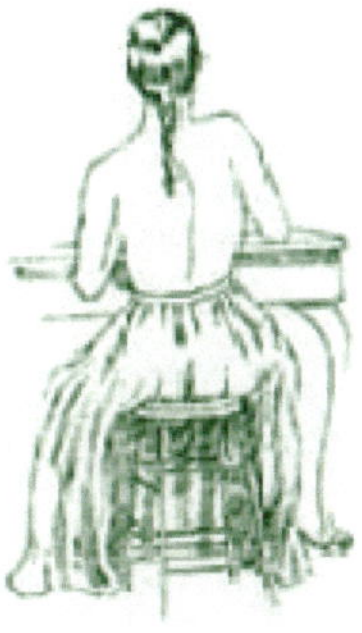

Desk Too High

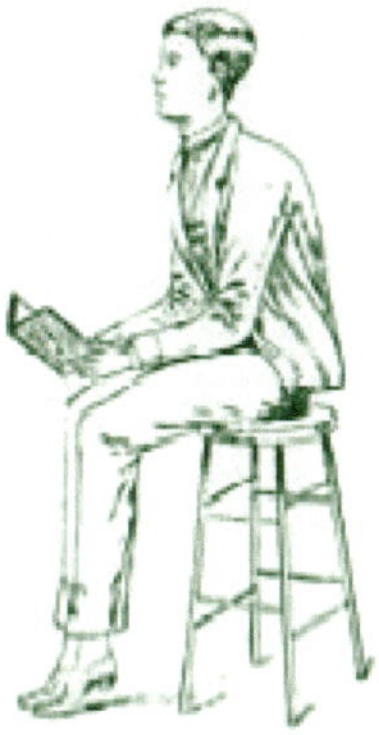

Seat Too High

When a man uses alcohol and tobacco, their effects upon the bones are not so apparent as are the effects upon the blood, the nerves, and other organs; but when the poisonous drugs are used by a growing child, their damaging influence is very plainly seen. A child who smokes cigars or cigarettes, or who uses strong alcoholic drinks, is likely to be so stunted that even his bones will not grow of a proper length and he will become dwarfed or deformed.

POINTS TO REMEMBER

1. To keep the bones healthy they must have plenty of healthful food.

2. The whole-grain preparations furnish the best food for the bones.

3. Bad positions and tight or poorly-fitting clothing my cause flat chests, round shoulders, and other deformities.

4. Tight or high-heeled shoes deform the feet and make the gait awkward.

5. The bones may be easily broken or put out of joint, or the ligaments may be torn by rough play.

6. Alcohol prevents healthy growth.

MUSCLES and HOW WE USE THEM

The Muscles–Where do people obtain the steaks and lamb-chops they eat? From the butcher, you will say; and the butcher gets them from the sheep and cattle which he kills. If you will clasp your arm you will notice that the bones are covered by a soft substance, the flesh. When the skin of an animal has been taken off, we can see that some of the flesh is white or yellow and some of it is red. The white or yellow flesh is fat. The red flesh is lean meat, and it is composed of muscles.

The Number of Muscles–We have about 639 different muscles in the body. They are arranged in such a way as to cover the bones and make the body round and beautiful. They are of different forms and sizes.

With a very few exceptions the muscles are arranged in pairs; that is, we have two alike of each form and size, one for each side of the body.

How a Muscle is Formed–If you will examine a piece of corned or salted beef which has been well boiled, you will notice that it seems to be made up of bundles of small fibers or threads of flesh. With a little care you can pick one of the small fibers into fine threads. Now, if you look at one of these under a microscope you find that it is made of still finer fibers, which are much smaller than the threads of a spider's web. One of these smallest threads is called a muscular fiber. Many thousands of muscular fibers are required to make a muscle.

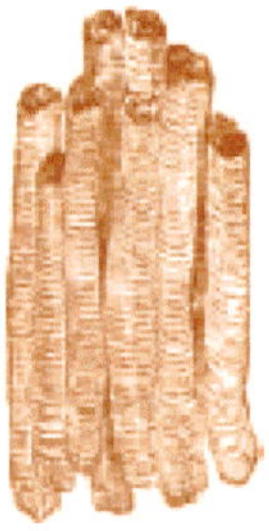

Muscular Fibers

Most of the muscles are fastened to the bones. Generally, one end is attached to one bone, and the other to another bone. Sometimes one end is fastened to a bone and the other to the skin or to other muscles.

The Tendons–Many of the muscles are not joined to the bones directly, but are made fast to them by means of firm cords called tendons. If you will place the thumb of your left hand upon the wrist of the right hand, and then work the fingers of the right hand, you may feel these cords moving underneath the skin.

What the Muscles Do–With the left hand grasp the right arm just in front of the elbow. Now shut the right hand tightly. Now open it. Repeat several times. The left hand feels something moving in the flesh. The motion is caused by the working of the muscles, which shorten and harden when they act.

All the movements of the body are made by means of muscles. When we move our hands, even when we close the mouth or the eyes, or make a wry face, we use the muscles. We could not speak, laugh, sing, or breathe without muscles.

Self-acting Muscles–Did you ever have a fit of sneezing or hiccupping? If you ever did, very likely you tried hard to stop but could not. Do you know why one cannot always stop sneezing or hiccupping when he desires to do so? It is because there are certain muscles in the body which do not act simply when we wish them to act, but when it is necessary that they should. The muscles which act when we sneeze or

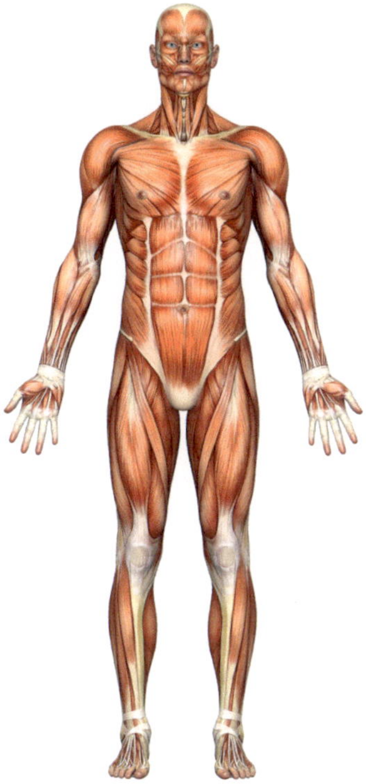

Muscles (Front View)

The stomach, the intestines, the blood vessels, and many other organs within the body have this kind of muscles. The work of these self-acting muscles is very wonderful indeed. Without it we could not live a moment. This knowledge should lead us to consider how dependent we are, each moment of our lives, upon the delicate machinery by which the most important work of our bodies is performed, and how particular we should be to keep it in good order by taking proper care of ourselves.

hiccup are of this kind. The arm and the hand do not act unless we wish them to do so. Suppose it were the same with the heart. We should have to stay awake all the while to keep it going, because it would not act when we were asleep. The same is true of our breathing. We breathe when we are asleep as well as when we are awake, because the breathing muscles work even when we do not think about them.

POINTS TO REMEMBER

1. The flesh, or lean meat, is composed of muscles.

2. There are about 639 muscles in the body.

3. Muscles are composed of many small threads called muscular fibers.

4. Many of the muscles are joined to the bones by strong white cords called tendons.

5. Muscular fibers can contract so as to lessen their length. It is in this way that the muscles perform their work.

6. All bodily motions are due to the action of the muscles.

7. Most of the muscles act only when we wish them to do so. Some muscles, however, act when it is necessary for them to do so, whether we will that they should act or not, and when we are asleep as well as when we are awake.

KEEPING MUSCLES HEALTHY

How to Make the Muscles Strong–With which hand can you lift the more? With the right hand or with the left? Why do you think you can lift more with the right hand than with the left? When an athlete throws a shot put or discus with his left arm, that arm becomes very large and strong. If we wish our muscles to grow large and strong, so that our bodies will be healthy and vigorous, we must take plenty of exercise.

Effects of Idleness–If a boy should carry one hand in his pocket all the time, and use only the other hand and arm, the idle arm would become small and weak, while the other would grow large and strong. Any part of the body which is not used will after a time become weak. Little boys and girls who do not take plenty of exercise are likely to become pale and puny. It is important that we should take the proper amount of exercise every day, just as we take our food and drink every day.

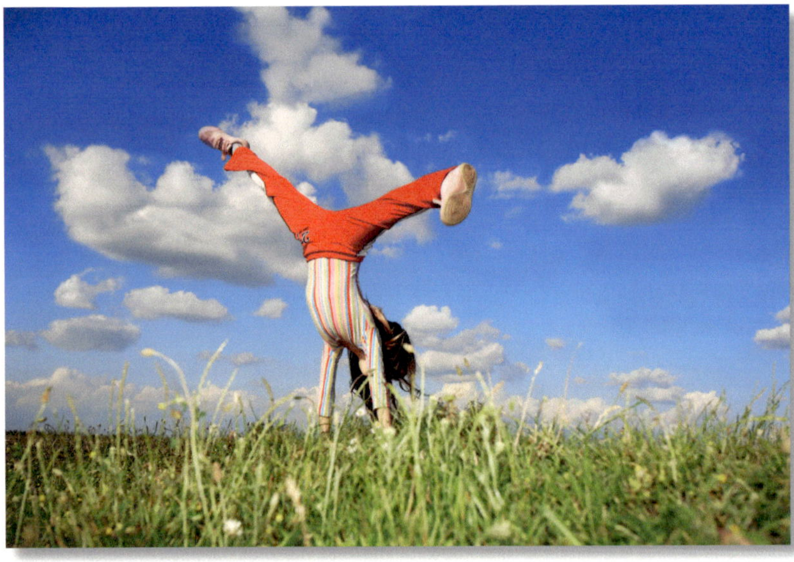

Healthful Exercise–Some kinds of play, and almost all kinds of work which children have to do, are good ways of taking exercise. A very good kind of exercise for little boys and girls is that found in running errands or doing chores about the house.

Food and Strength–A great part of our food goes to nourish the muscles. Some foods make us strong, while others do not. Plain foods, such as bread, meat, potatoes, and milk, are good for the muscles; but cakes and pies, and things which are not food, such as mustard, pepper, and spices, do not give us strength, and are likely to do us harm.

Over-Exertion–We ought not to exert ourselves too much in lifting heavy weights, or trying to do things which are too hard for us. Sometimes the muscles are permanently injured in this way.

The Clothing–We ought not to wear our clothing so tight as to press hard upon any part of the body. If we do, it will cause the muscles of that part to become weak. If the clothing is worn tight about the waist, great mischief is often done. The lungs cannot expand properly, the stomach and liver are pressed out of shape, and the internal organs are crowded out of their proper places.

Tight Shoes–People are often made very lame from wearing tight shoes. Their muscles cannot act properly, and their feet grow out of shape. In China, it was once fashionable for rich ladies to have small feet, and they tied them up in cloths

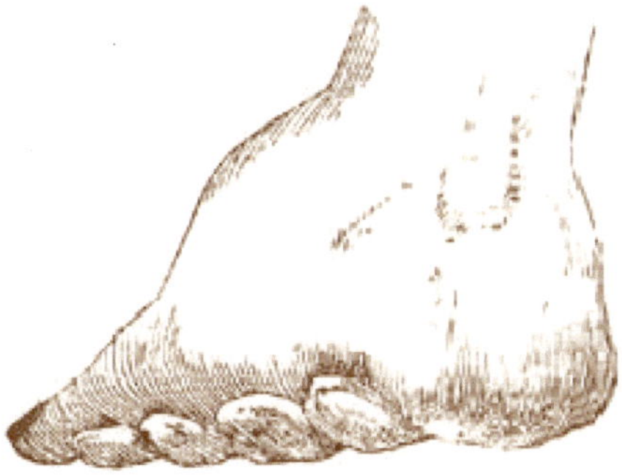

so that they would not grow. The foot was squeezed out of shape. Here is a picture of a foot which has been treated in this way. It does not look much like a human foot, does it? A woman who has such feet finds it so difficult to walk that she has to be carried about much of the time. Do you not think it is very wrong and foolish to treat the feet so badly? You will say, "Yes;" but the Chinese woman thought it a great deal worse to lace the clothing tight about the body so as to make the waist small as American women once did.

Effects of Alcohol upon the Muscles–When an intemperate man takes a glass of strong drink, it makes him feel strong; but when he tries to lift, or to do any kind of hard work, he cannot lift so much nor work so hard as he could have done without the alcohol. This is because alcohol poisons the muscles and makes them weak.

Effects of Drunkenness–When a man or woman has become addicted to strong drink, their muscles become partly paralyzed, so that he cannot walk as steadily or speak as readily or as clearly as before. Their fingers are clumsy, and their movements uncertain. If he or she is an artist or a jeweler, they cannot do as fine work as when they are sober. When a person gets very drunk, he or she is for a time completely paralyzed, so that they cannot walk or move, and seem almost dead.

If you had a good horse that had carried you a long way in a carriage, and you wanted to travel farther, what would you do if the horse were so tired that he kept stopping in the road? Would you let him rest and give him some water to drink and some nice hay and oats to eat, or would you strike him hard with a whip to make him go faster? If you should whip him he would act as though he were not tired at all, but do you think the whip would make him strong, as rest and hay and oats would?

When a tired person takes alcohol, it acts like a whip; it makes every part of the body work faster and harder than it ought to work, and thus wastes the one's strength and makes them

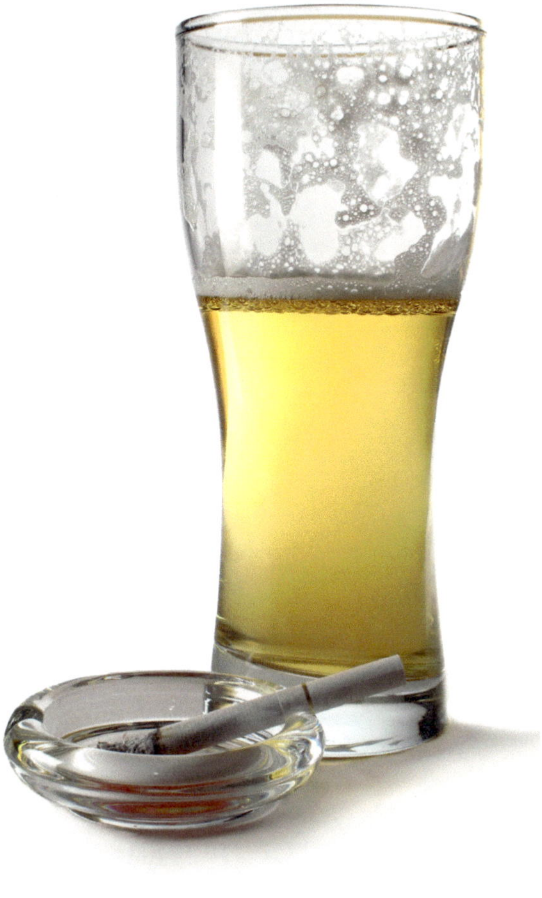

weaker, although for a little while the nerves are made stupid, so that the person does not know that they are tired and ought to rest.

When you grow up to be a man and woman you will want to have strong muscles. So you must be careful not to give alcohol a chance to injure them. If you never taste it in any form you will be sure to suffer no harm from it.

Effects of Tobacco on the Muscles–Boys and girls who smoke cigars or cigarettes, or who chew tobacco, are not likely to grow up to be strong and healthy adults. They do not have plump and rosy cheeks and strong muscles like other children.

The evil effect of tobacco upon children is now so well known that in the United States laws have been made which do not allow alcohol or tobacco to be sold or given to children. When a child smokes, they rob their body of its vigor, and allow tobacco to steal away from them the strength they will need when they become an adult.

Tea and Coffee–Strong caffeinated tea and coffee, while by no means so bad as alcohol and tobacco, may make us weak and sick. A person who drinks strong tea or coffee feels less tired while at work than if they had not taken it, but they are more tired afterwards. So you see that tea and coffee are also whips, small whips we might call them, and yet they really act in the same way as do other narcotics and stimulants. They make a person feel stronger than they really are, and thus they are led to use more strength than they can afford to do.

POINTS TO REMEMBER

1. We must use the muscles to make them grow large and strong.

2. Exercise should be taken regularly.

3. Exercise makes the muscles strong, the body beautiful, the lungs active, the heart vigorous, and the whole body healthy.

4. Things we ought not to do: To run or play hard just before or after eating; to strain our muscles by lifting too heavy weights; to exercise so violently as to get out of breath; to lie, sit, stand, or walk in a cramped position, or awkward manner; to wear the clothing so tight as to press hard upon the muscles.

5. Good food is necessary to make the muscles strong and healthy.

6. Alcohol makes the muscles weak, although at first it makes us feel stronger.

7. A child who uses tobacco will not grow as strong and well as one who does not.

8. The use of caffeinated tea and coffee may injure the muscles.

HOW WE FEEL and THINK

How We Think–With what part of the body do we think? You will at once say that we think with the head; but we do not think with the whole head. Some parts of the head we use for other purposes, as the mouth to eat and speak with, and the nose to smell and breathe with. The part we think with is inside of the skull, safely placed in a little room at the top and back part of the head. Do you remember the name of this organ which fills the hollow place inside of the skull? We learned some time ago that it is called the brain. It is with the brain that we study and remember and reason. So the brain is one of the most important organs in our body, and we must try to learn all we can about it.

The Brain–You cannot see and examine your own brain because it is shut up in the skull; but perhaps you can find the brain of a sheep or a calf at the meat market. The brain of one of these animals looks very nearly like your own.

The Large Brain and the Small Brain–In examining a brain we should notice first of all that there are really two brains, a large brain and a small brain. The large brain is in the top and front of the skull, and the small one lies beneath the back part of the larger one, If we look again we shall see that each brain is divided in the middle into a right and a left half. Each half is, in fact, a complete brain, so that we really have two pairs of brains.

Brain Cells–The brain is a curious organ of a grayish color outside and white inside. It is soft, almost like jelly, and this is why it is placed so carefully in a strong, bony box. If we should put a little piece of the brain under a microscope, we should find that it is made up of a great number of very small objects called nerve or

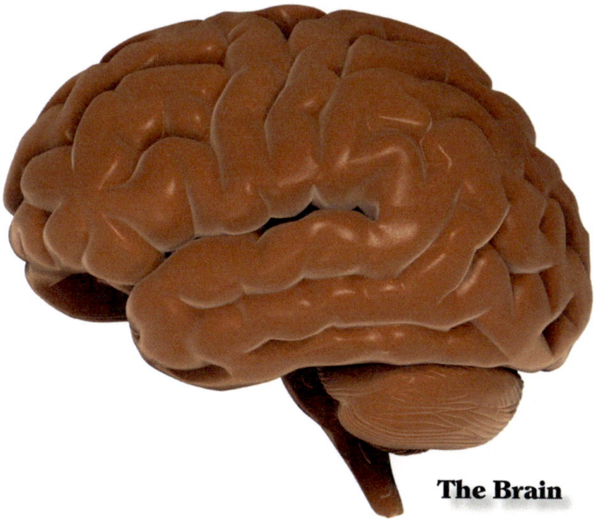

The Brain

brain cells. In the illustration you can see some of these brain cells.

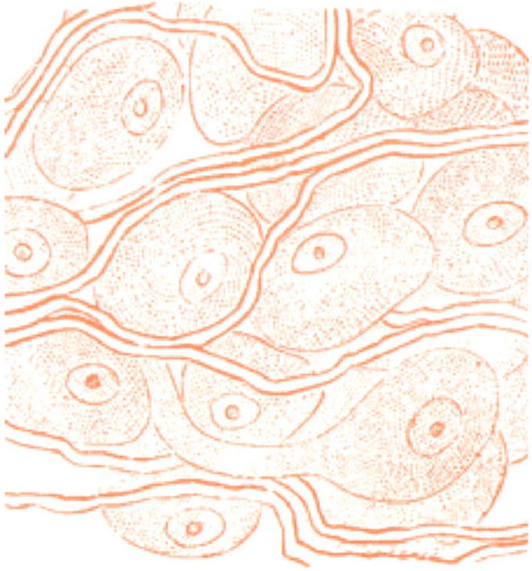

Brain Cells

The Nerves–Each cell has one or more branches. Some of the branches are joined to the branches of other cells so as to unite the cells together, just as children take hold of one another's hands. Other branches are drawn out very long.

The long branches are such slender threads that a great number of them together would not be as large as a fine silk thread. A great many of these fine nerve threads are bound up in little bundles which look like white cords. These are called nerves.

The nerves branch out from the brain through openings in the skull, and go to every part of the body. Every little muscle fiber, the heart, the stomach, the lungs, the liver, even the bones–all have nerves coming to them from the brain. So you see that the brain is not wholly shut up in the skull, because its cells have slender branches running into all parts of the body; and thus the brain itself is really in every part of the body, though we usually speak of it as being entirely in the skull.

The Spinal Cord–There are a number of small holes in the skull through which the nerves pass out, but most of the nerves are bound up in one large bundle and pass out through an opening at the back part of the skull and runs downward through a long canal in the spinal column. This bundle of nerves forms the spinal cord. The spinal cord contains cells also, like those of the brain. It is really a continuation of the brain down through the spinal column.

Nerves from the Spinal Cord–The spinal cord gives off branches of nerves which go to the arms, the chest, the legs, and other parts. One of the branches which goes to the hand runs along the back side of the arm, passing over the elbow. If we happen to strike the elbow against some sharp object, we sometimes hit this nerve. When we do so, the under side of the arm and the little finger feel very numb and strange. This is why you call this part of the elbow the "funny" or "crazy bone." The cells of the spinal cord also send out branches to the body and to other cells in the brain.

How We Feel–If we cut or burn ourselves we suffer pain. Can you tell why it hurts us to prick the flesh with a pin, or to pinch or burn or bruise it? It is because the flesh contains a great many nerve branches from the brain. When we hurt the skin or the flesh, in any way, these nerves are injured. There are so many of these little nerves in the flesh and skin that we cannot put the finest needle into the flesh without hurting some of them.

The Use of Pain–It is not pleasant for us to have pain, but if the nerves gave us no pain when we are hurt we might get our limbs burned or frozen and know nothing about it until too late to save them.

Nerves of Feeling–We have different kinds of nerves of feeling. Those we have learned about feel pain. Others feel objects. If you take a marble or a pencil in the hand you know what it is by the feeling of the object. This kind of feeling is called the sense of touch.

There are other nerves of feeling by means of which we are able to hear, see, taste, and smell, of which we shall learn in another lesson. Besides these we have nerves which tell us whether objects are cold or hot, and heavy or light. Nerves of feeling also tell us when we are hungry, or thirsty, or tired, and when we need more air to breathe.

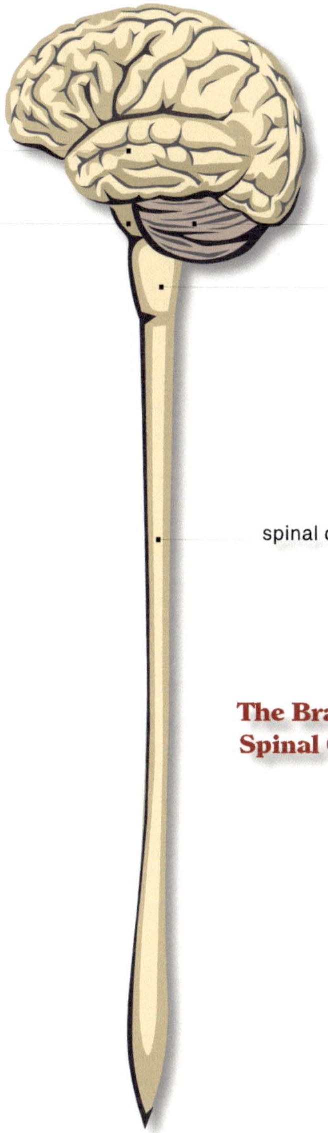

The Brain and Spinal Cord

Nerves of Work–There are other nerves which are made just like the nerves of feeling, but which do not feel. These nerves have a very different use. They come from cells in the brain which have charge of the different kinds of work done in the body, and they send their branches to the parts which do the work; hence we call them nerves of work.

One set of cells sends nerve messages, or impulses, to the heart, and these make it go fast or slow as is necessary. Another sends nerve impulses to the liver, stomach, and other digestive organs, and causes them to do their part in the digestion of the food. Other cells send nerve impulses to the muscles and make them act when we wish them to do so. Thus you see how very useful the brain and nerves are. They keep all the different parts of the body working together in harmony, just like a well-trained army, or a great number of workmen building a block of houses. Without the brain and nerves the body would be just like an army without a commander, or a lot of workmen without an overseer.

How We Use the Nerves–If you happen to touch your hand to a hot stove, what takes place? You will say that your arm pulls the hand away. Do you know why? Let us see. The nerves of feeling in the hand tell the nerve cells in the brain from which they come that the hand is being burned. The cells which feel cannot do anything for the hand, but some of their branches run over to another part of the brain, which sends nerve impulses down to the muscles of the arm. These cells, through their nerve branches, cause the muscles to contract. The cells of feeling ask the cells which have charge of the muscles to make the muscles of the arm pull the hand away, which they do very quickly.

So you see the nerves are very much like telephone wires. By means of them the brain finds out all about what is happening in the body, and sends out its orders to the various organs, which may be called its servants.

An Experiment–A man once tried an experiment which seemed very cruel. He took a dove and cut open its skull and took out its large brain. What do you think the effect was? The dove did not die at once, as you would expect.

It lived for some time, but it did not know anything. It did not know when it was hungry, and would not eat or drink unless the food or water was placed in its mouth. If a man gets a blow on his head, so hard as to break his skull, the large brain is often hurt so badly that its cells cannot work, and so the man is in the same condition as the poor dove. He does not know anything. He cannot think or talk, and lies as though he were asleep.

By these and many other facts we know that the large brain is the part with which we remember, think, and reason. It is the seat of the mind. We go to sleep because the large brain is tired and cannot work any longer. We stop thinking when we are sound asleep, but sometimes we do not sleep soundly, and then the large brain works a little and we dream.

What the Little Brain Does–The little brain[1] thinks too, but it does not do the same kind of thinking as the large brain. We may use our arms and legs and many other parts when we wish to do so; and if we do not care to use them we may allow them to remain quiet. This is not the case with some other organs. It is necessary, for example, that the heart, the lungs, and many other organs of the body should keep at work all the time. If the large brain had to attend to all of these different kinds of work besides thinking about what we see, hear, and read, and other things which we do, it would have too much work to do, and would not be able to do it all well. Besides, the large brain sometimes falls asleep. So the large brain lets the little brain do the kinds of work which have to be attended to all the time, and the little brain keeps steadily at work when we are asleep as well as when we are awake.

What the Spinal Cord Does–If you tickle a person's foot when they are asleep, they will pull it up just as they would if awake, only not quite so quickly. What do you suppose makes the muscles of the leg contract when the brain is asleep and does not know that the foot is being tickled? And here is another curious fact. When you walk you do not have to think about every step you take. You can talk or read but your legs walk right along all the time, and without your thinking about them. Can you tell how?

It would be too much trouble for the large brain to stop to think every time we step, and the little brain has work enough to do in taking care of the heart and lungs and other organs, without keeping watch of the feet when we are asleep, so as to pull them up if some mischievous person tickles them. So God puts a few nerve cells in the spinal cord which can do a certain easy kind of thinking. When we do things over and over a great many times, these cells, after a time, learn to do them without the help of the large brain. This is the way a piano player becomes so expert. The pianist does not have to think all the time where each finger is to go. After the tunes have been played a great many times, the spinal cord knows them so well that it makes the hands play them almost without any effort of the large brain.

[1] For the sake of brevity and clearness the author has included under the term "little brain" the *medulla oblongata* as well as the *cerebellum*.

POINTS TO REMEMBER

1. The part of the body with which we think is the brain.

2. The brain is found filling the hollow place in the skull.

3. There are two brains, the large brain and the small brain.

4. Each brain is divided into two equal and complete halves, thus making two pairs of brains.

5. The brain is largely made up of very small objects called nerve or brain cells.

6. The nerve cells send out very fine branches which form the nerves.

7. The nerve branches or fibers run to every part of the body. They pass out from the brain to the rest of the body through a number of openings in the skull.

8. Most of the nerve branches pass out through a large opening at the back of the skull, in one large bundle called the spinal cord.

9. The spinal cord runs down through a canal in the backbone, and all along gives off branches to the various parts of the body.

10. It gives us pain to prick or hurt the flesh in any way, because when we do so we injure some of the little nerve branches of the brain cells.

11. When we suffer, we really feel a pain in the brain. We know this because if a nerve is cut in two, we may hurt the part to which it goes without giving any pain.

12. We have different kinds of nerves of feeling.

13. There are other nerves besides those of feeling. These are nerves of work.

14. The nerves of work have charge of the heart, the lungs, the muscles, the liver, the stomach, and every part of the body which can work or act.

15. The brain and nerves control the body and make all the different parts work together in harmony, just as a general controls an army.

16. The brain uses the nerves very much as a man uses the telephone wires.

17. With the large brain we remember, think, and reason.

18. The little brain does the simple kind of thinking, by means of which the heart, lungs, and other vital organs are kept at work even when we are asleep.

19. The spinal cord does a still more simple kind of work. It enables us to walk and to do other familiar acts without using the large brain to think every moment just what we are doing.

A HEALTHY BRAIN and NERVES

Uses of the Brain–What do you think a boy or girl would be good for without any brain or nerves? Such a boy or girl could not see, hear, feel, talk, run about, or play, and would not know any more than a cabbage or a potato knows. If the brain or nerves are sick, they cannot work well, and so are not worth as much as when they are healthy.

The Brain Sympathizes with Other Organs–Did you ever have a headache? Did you feel happy and good-natured when your head ached hard, and could you study and play as well as when you are well? It is very important that we should keep our brain and nerves healthy, and to do this we must take good care of the stomach and all other organs, because the brain sympathizes with them when they are sick.

We Must Have Pure Air–How do you feel when a room is too warm and close? Do you not feel dull and sleepy and so stupid that you can hardly think? This is because the brain needs good, pure blood to enable it to work well. So we must always be careful to have plenty of pure air to breathe.

We Should Exercise the Brain–What do we do when we want to strengthen our muscles? We make them work hard every day, do we not? The exercise makes them grow large and strong. It is just the same with our brains. If we study hard and learn our lessons well, then our brains grow strong, and study becomes easy. But if we only half study, and do not learn our lessons perfectly, then the study does not do our brains very much good.

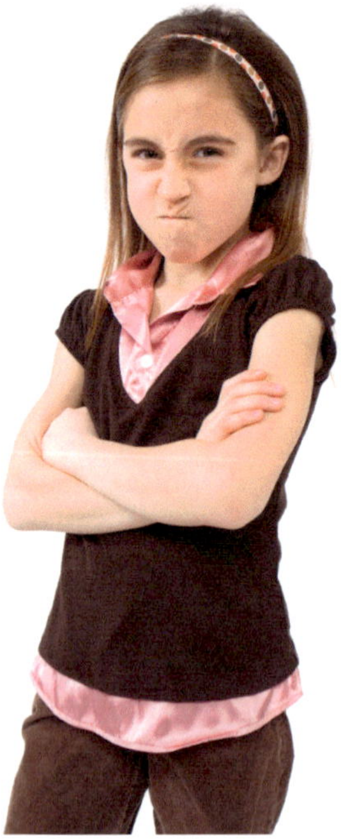

We Should Take Muscular Exercise–When you get tired of study, an hour's play, or exercise of some sort, rests you and makes you feel brighter, so that you can learn more easily. This is because exercise is necessary to make the blood circulate well. It will then carry out the worn out particles and supply the brain and nerves with fresh, pure blood. So the same exercise which makes our muscles strong makes our brains healthier also.

We Should Be Careful of Our Diet–We ought to eat plenty of good, simple food, such as milk, fruits, grains, and vegetables. It is not well for children to eat freely of meat, as it is very stimulating and likely to excite the brain and make the nerves irritable. Mustard, pepper, and all hot sauces and spices have a tendency to injure the brain and nerves.

We Should Allow the Brain to Rest at the Proper Time–When we are tired and sleepy we cannot think well, and cannot remember what we learn if we try to study. If we have plenty of sleep, free from bad or exciting dreams, we awake in the morning rested and refreshed, because while we have been asleep our body has put the brain and nerves in good repair for us. We ought not to stay up late at night. We should not eat late or heavy suppers, as this will prevent our sleeping well.

We Ought Not to Allow Ourselves to Become Too Angry–When a person flies into a passion he does his brain and nerves great harm. It is really dangerous to get too angry. Persons have dropped dead instantly in a fit of anger.

We Should Shun Bad Habits–Bad habits are very hard to give up, and hence we should be careful to avoid them. When a child learns to swear, or to use slang phrases, the brain after a while will make him swear or use bad words without even thinking. In a similar manner other bad habits are acquired.

POINTS TO REMEMBER

1. A person without a brain or nerves would be of no more account than a vegetable.

2. When the brain or nerves are sick they cannot perform their duties properly.

3. To keep the brain and nerves in good health, we must take good care of the stomach and all other important organs of the body.

4. There are many things which we may do to keep the brain and nerves strong and well.

5. The brain needs pure blood, and so we must be careful to breathe pure air.

6. The brain gets strength by exercise, just as the muscles do. Hence, study is healthful, and makes the brain strong.

7. A good memory is very necessary, but we should not try to remember everything.

8. It is very important that we learn how to observe things closely.

9. Exercise in the open air rests and clears the brain by helping the blood to circulate.

10. Plenty of wholesome and simple food is necessary to keep the brain and nerves in good health. Spices, condiments, and rich foods in general are stimulating and harmful.

11. Plenty of sleep is needed to rest the brain and nerves.

12. It is dangerous to become very angry.

13. We should be careful to avoid forming bad habits of any sort, as they are hard to break, and often adhere to one through life.

POISONING the BRAIN and NERVES

Drunkenness–Did you ever see a man who was drunk? If you live in a city it is very likely that you have. How did the drunken man behave? Perhaps he was noisy and silly. Perhaps he was angry and tried to pick a quarrel with some one.

What made the man drunk? You say whiskey, but it may have been wine, or beer, or hard cider that he drank. Anything that contains alcohol will make a man drunk, for it is the alcohol which does all the mischief.

The Whiskey Flush–You can almost always tell when a man has been drinking, even when he has not taken enough to make him drunk. You know by his flushed face and red eyes. When a man's face blushes from the use of alcohol, his whole body blushes at the same time. His muscles, his lungs, and his liver blush; his brain and spinal cord blush also.

When a man has taken just enough alcohol to make his face blush a little, the extra amount of blood in the brain makes him think and talk more lively, and he is very jolly and cheerful. This makes many people think that alcohol does them good. But if we notice what a man says when he is excited by alcohol, we shall find that his remarks are often silly and reckless. He says very unwise and foolish things, for which he feels sorry when he becomes sober.

Alcohol Paralyzes–How does a drunken man walk? Let us see why he staggers. When a man takes a certain amount of alcohol his small brain and spinal cord become partly paralyzed, so that they cannot do their duty well; and so, when he tries to walk he reels and stumbles along, often falling down, and sometimes hurting himself very much. The fact is that the alcohol has put his spinal cord and small brain to sleep so that he cannot make his legs do what he wants them to do. Now, if still more alcohol is taken the whole brain becomes paralyzed, and then the man is so nearly dead that we say he is "dead drunk." It is exceedingly dangerous to become dead drunk, as the brain

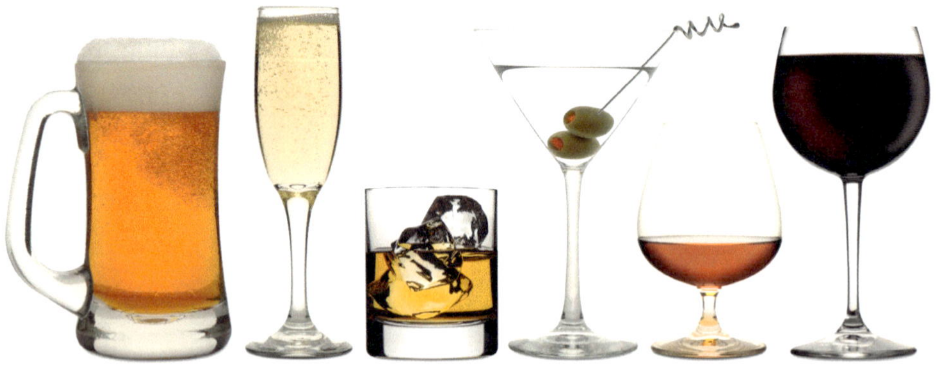

may be so completely paralyzed that it will not recover.

A small amount of alcohol does not make a man dead drunk, but it poisons and paralyzes his brain and nerves just according to the quantity he takes.

If a person holds a little alcohol in his mouth for a few moments, the tongue and cheeks feel numb. This is because the alcohol paralyzes them so that they cannot feel or taste. When taken into the stomach it has much the same kind of effect upon the nerves of the whole body.

Alcohol a Deceiver–A hungry man takes a drink of whiskey and benumbs the nerves of his stomach so that he does not feel hungry. Alcohol puts to sleep the sentinels which God has set in the body to warn us of danger. A man who is cold takes alcohol and feels warm, though he is really colder. He lies down in his false comfort and freezes to death. A tired man takes his glass of grog and feels rested and strong, though he is really weaker than before. A poor man gets drunk and feels so rich that he spends what little money he has. The alcohol paralyzes his judgment and steals away his good sense. Thus alcohol is always a deceiver.

Delirium Tremens (De-leer'-ee-um Tre'-mens)–When a man takes strong alcohol regularly he very soon injures his brain and nerves so that they do not get quiet, as they should, at night, and he does not sleep well. He has frightful dreams. He sees all sorts of wild animals and horrid shapes in his dreams. Perhaps you have sometimes had such dreams from eating late suppers or indigestible food.

Did you ever have a dream when you were awake? If a man drinks a great deal he is likely to have a terrible disease known as delirium tremens, in which he sees the same frightful things when he is wide awake that he dreams about when he is asleep. This is one of the terrible effects of alcohol upon the brain and nerves.

Alcohol Paralysis–You have seen how a drunken man staggers when he walks. Did you ever see a man who walked just as though he were drunk when he was really sober? This is because a part of the brain or spinal cord has been permanently injured or paralyzed. Alcohol is not the only cause of this disease, and so you must not think every person who staggers is or has been a drunkard; but alcohol is a very frequent cause of paralysis.

Effects of Alcohol Upon the Mind and Character–When a man is under the influence of alcohol is his character good or bad? Is a man likely to be good, or to be bad, when he is drunk or excited by drink? Most men behave badly when they are drunk, and after they have been drunk a great many times they often behave badly all the time. A great many of the men who are shut up in prisons would not have been sent there if they had never learned to drink.

A Legacy–Do you know what a legacy is? If your father should die and leave to you a fine house or farm, or money in the bank, or books, or horses, or any other kind of property to have for your own, it would be a legacy. When a person gets anything in this way from a parent we say that he inherits it.

We inherit a great many things besides houses and lands and other kinds of property. For instance, perhaps you remember hearing some one say that you have eyes and hair the same color as your mother's, and that your nose and chin are like your father's. So you have inherited the color of your hair and eyes from your mother and the shape of your chin and nose from your father.

The Alcohol Legacy–The inside of a child's head is just as much like their parents' as the outside of it. In other words, we inherit our brains just as we do our faces. So, if a man spoils his brain with alcohol and gets an alco-

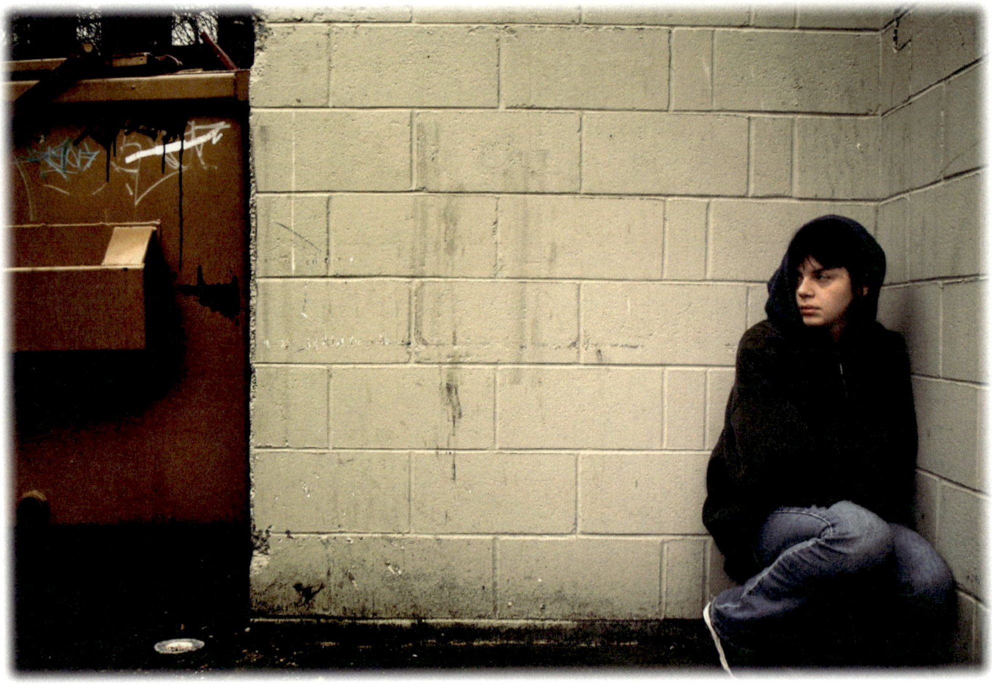

hol appetite, his children will be likely to have unhealthy brains and an appetite for alcohol also, and may become drunkards. Is not that a dreadful kind of legacy to inherit?

Some children whose parents drank too much alcohol cannot talk, or read, or sing, and do not know enough to take proper care of themselves. This is one of the bad legacies which drunken parents sometimes leave to their children.

Effects of Tobacco on the Brain and Nerves–The effects of tobacco upon the brain and nerves are much the same as those of alcohol. Tobacco, like alcohol, is a narcotic. It benumbs and paralyzes the nerves, and it is by this means that it obtains such an influence over those who use it.

The hand of a person who uses tobacco often becomes so unsteady that he can scarcely write. Do you know what makes it so unsteady? It is because the cells which send nerves to the muscles of the hand are diseased. When a person has a trembling hand you say they are nervous. If you feel the pulse you will find that it does not beat steadily and regularly as it ought to do. The heart is nervous and trembles just the same as the muscles do. This shows that the tobacco has poisoned the cells in the brain which regulate the heart.

Wise physicians will tell you that one reason why tobacco is bad for children is that it hurts their brains so that they cannot learn well, and do not become as useful and successful as they might be.

Tobacco Leads to Vice–Boys and girls who use tobacco are more liable to get into company with children who have other bad habits, and so are apt to become bad in many other ways. The use of tobacco often makes adults want strong drink, and thus leads to drunkenness. If you wish to grow up with a steady hand, a strong heart, and a good character you will never touch tobacco.

Effects of Tea and Coffee on the Nerves–People who use strong caffeinated tea and coffee are often inclined to be nervous. This shows that strong tea and coffee, like alcohol and tobacco, are very injurious to the nerves.

Other Drugs–There are several drugs which are given by physicians to relieve pain or to produce sleep. They are sometimes helpful, but their use is very dangerous. The danger is that, after a person has used these medicines a little while, will continue to use them. If a person takes a poisonous drug every time they have a little pain, they will soon form the habit of using it, and may never break it off. There are many thousands of people who use drugs more than advised by their physicians, and they are very much injured by it in mind and body. The mind becomes dull and stupid and the body weak and feeble. No medicine of this sort should ever be taken unless prescribed by a physician.

POINTS TO REMEMBER

1. In order to be well and useful we must keep the brain and nerves healthy.

2. To keep the brain healthy we need plenty of pure air to breathe; proper exercise of the brain by study; sufficient exercise of the muscles in play and work; plenty of good food to make pure blood; a proper amount of rest and sleep.

3. There are several things we ought not to do. We should not read or study too much. We should not allow ourselves to become too excited or angry. We should avoid learning bad habits.

4. Alcohol paralyzes the brain and nerves.

5. Alcohol deceives a person who takes it by making them feel strong when they are weak; warm when they are cold; rich when they are poor; well when they are sick.

6. Alcohol makes people make bad decisions. Most people who commit crimes are people who use alcohol.

7. The effects of tobacco upon the brain and nerves are much the same as those of alcohol. Tobacco is very injurious to the mind.

8. Tobacco using often leads children to drunkenness and other vices.

9. The use of misuse of prescription drugs produces even worse effects than the use of alcohol or tobacco.

HOW WE HEAR, TASTE, SMELL and FEEL

The Senses–We have five senses–hearing, seeing, smelling, tasting, and feeling. These are called special senses because they are very different from each other. They also differ from the general sense of feeling by means of which we feel pain when any part is hurt.

Organs of the Special Senses–Each of the special senses has a special set of nerves and also special cells in the brain which have charge of them. We say that we see with our eyes, hear with our ears, feel with our fingers, etc.; but, really, we see, hear, taste, and smell in the brain just as we feel in the brain. The eyes, ears, nose, and other organs of the special senses are the instruments by means of which the brain sees, hears, smells, etc.

Sound and the Vibrations which it Causes–All sounds are made by vibrations of objects. Sounds cause objects to vibrate or tremble. A loud sound sometimes jars a whole house, while other sounds are so gentle and soft that we cannot feel them in the same way that we feel loud sounds. But God has made for us an ingenious organ by means of which we can feel these very fine vibrations as well as loud ones. We call this organ the ear.

The Ear–The part of the ear which we can see is shaped somewhat like a trumpet. The small opening near the middle of the ear leads into a canal or tube which extends into the head about an inch. At the inner end there is a curious little chamber. This is called the drum of the ear, because between it and the canal of the ear there is stretched a thin membrane like the head of a drum sometimes called the ear drum, or the tympanic (tim-pa´-nik) membrane . This canal is also called the middle ear.

Bones of the Ear–Within the drum of the ear there are three curious little bones which are joined together so as to make a complete chain, reaching from the drumhead to the other side of the drum. The last bone fits into a little hole which leads into another curious chamber. This chamber, which is called the inner ear, is filled with fluid, and in this fluid the nerve of hearing is spread out. A part of the inner ear looks very much like a snail shell.

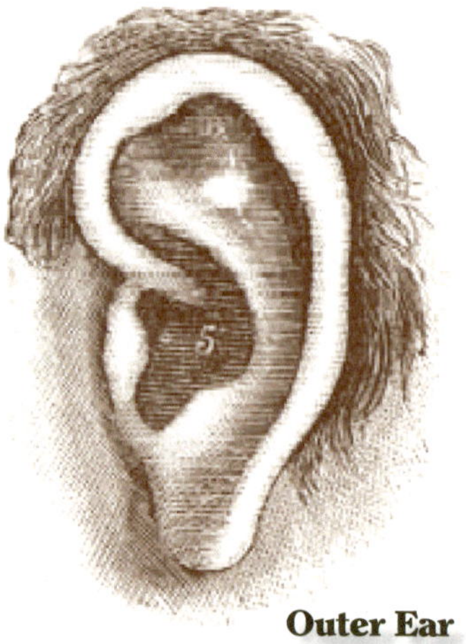

Outer Ear

How We Hear–Scratch with a pin upon one end of a long wooden pole. Have some one listen with the ear placed close against the other end of the pole. He will tell you that he hears the scratching of the pin very plainly. This is because the scratching vibrates the ear and especially the drumhead, which vibrates just as the head of a drum does when it is beaten with a drumstick. When the drumhead vibrates it moves the bones of the ear, called the malleus (mal´-ee-us), stapes (stay´-peez), and incus (in´-kus). These bones send vibrations to the cochlea (coke´-lee-uh). The cochlea translates the

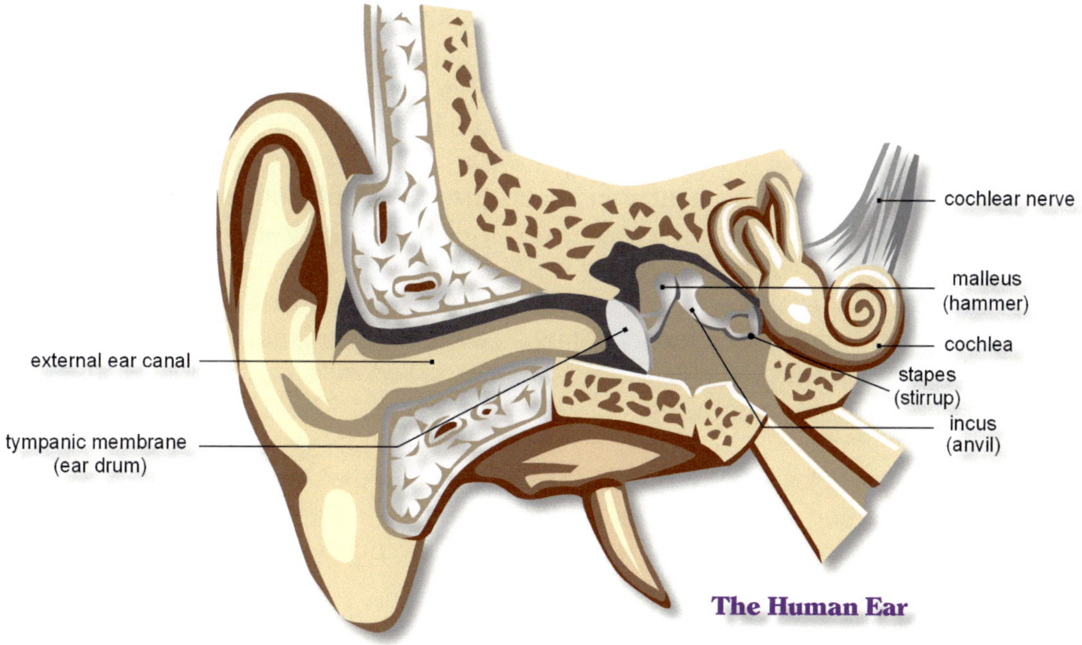

The Human Ear

vibrations for the cochlear nerve, which then sends impulses to the brain which we hear as sound. We hear all sounds in the same way, only most sounds come to the ear through the air.

How to Keep the Ears Healthy–The ears are very delicate organs and must be carefully treated. The following things about the care of the ears should never be forgotten:

(1) Never use a pin, toothpick, or any other sharp instrument to clean out the ear. There is great danger that the tympanic membrane will be torn, and thus the hearing will be injured. Neither is it ever necessary to use an ear-spoon to remove the wax. Working at the ear causes more wax to form.

(2) Do not allow cold water to enter the ear or a cold wind to blow directly into it.

(3) If anything accidentally gets into the ear, do not work at it, but hold the head over to one side while water is made to run in from a syringe. If an insect has gone into the ear, have an adult pour in a little mineral oil. This will kill the insect or make it come out.

(4) Never allow loud music or noisy machines to be close to the ear; it is better to wear ear plugs in these instances to protect the ear. Never shout into another person's ear. Otherwise, the ear may be greatly injured.

(5) Boxing the ears is likely to produce deafness, and ought never to be done.

The Eye–The eye is one of the most wonderful organs in the whole body. It enables us to know what is going on at some distance from us, and to enjoy many beautiful things which our sense of hearing and other senses can tell us nothing about. It also enables us to read. Let us learn how this wonderful organ is made.

The Eyeball–Looking at the eye, we see first a round part which rolls in different directions. This is the eyeball. We see only the front side of the eyeball as it fits into a hollow in the skull. Being thus in a safe place, it is not likely to get hurt.

The eyeball is mostly filled with a clear substance very much like jelly. It is so clear that the light can shine through it just as easily as it can shine through water.

The Pupil–If you look sharply at the eyeball you will see a small black hole just in the center. This is a little window which lets the light into the inside of the eyeball. We call this the pupil. Just around the pupil is a colored ring called the iris (eye´-ris) which gives the eye its color. We say a person has blue or brown or gray eyes according as this ring is blue or brown or gray. The iris is a kind of curtain for the window of the eye.

If you observe the pupil closely, you will see that it is sometimes larger and sometimes smaller. If you look at the light the pupil is small; if you turn away from the light the pupil grows larger at once. This is because the iris closes when in a bright light and opens in the darkness. It does this of itself without our thinking about it. In this way the eye is protected from too strong a light, which would do it great harm.

If you look a little sidewise at the eyeball, you will see that the iris has something in front of it which is clear as glass. It is about the shape of a watch crystal, only very much smaller. It is called the cornea (cor´-nee-uh). This is to the eye what the glass is to the windows of a house. It closes the opening in the front of the eyeball and yet lets the light shine in.

The White of the Eye–The white of the eye is a tough, firm membrane which encloses the eyeball and keeps it in a round shape.

The Lens–Do you know what a lens is? Perhaps you do not know it by this name, but you are familiar with the glasses which people sometimes wear to help their eyes. The glasses in the frames are called lenses. Well, there is something in the eye almost exactly like one of these lenses, only smaller. It is also called a lens. The lens is placed in the eyeball just behind the pupil.

The Nerves of Sight–But a person might have an eyeball with all the parts we have learned about and yet not be able to see. Can you tell what more is needed? There must be a nerve. This nerve comes from some little nerve cells in the brain and enters the eyeball at the back of the eye; there it is spread out on the inside of the black lining of the white of the eye. This is called the optical (op´-tuh-kuhl) nerve. The black lining is called the retina (ret´-uh-nuh). The retina is made of special nerve cells connected to the optical nerve. Some of these cells are called rods and cones, because of how they are shaped. These rods and cones receive the light that passes through the lens and create impulses that travel through the optical nerve into the brain. The brain turns these impulses into the images that we call sight.

The Eyelids–Now we know all that it is necessary for us to learn about the eyeball, so let us notice some other parts about the eye. First

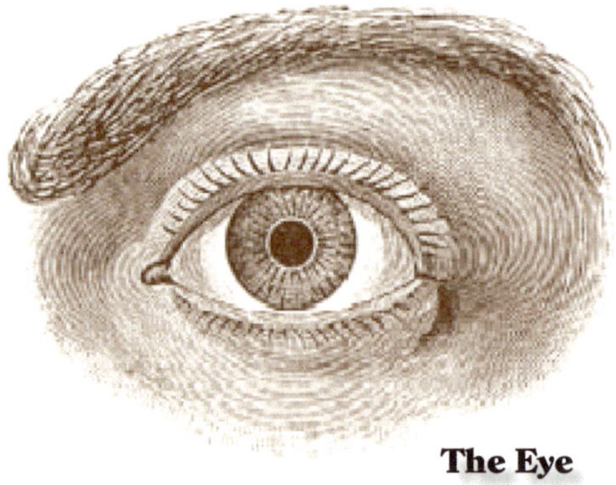

The Eye

there are the eyelids. They are little folds of skin fringed with hairs, which we can shut up so as to cover the eyeball and keep out the light when we want to sleep or when we are in danger of getting dust or smoke into the eye. The hairs placed along the edge of the lids help to keep the dust out when the eyes are open.

The Eyebrows–The row of hairs placed above the eye is called the eyebrow. Like the eyelids, the eyebrows catch some substances which might fall into the eye, and they also serve to run off the perspiration and keep it out of the eyes.

The Tear Gland–Do you know where the tears come from? There is a little gland snugly placed away in the socket of the eye just above the eyeball, which makes tears in the same way that the salivary glands make saliva. It is called the tear gland. The gland usually makes just enough tears to keep the eye moist. There are times when it makes more than enough, as when something gets into the eye, or when we suffer pain or feel unhappy. Then the tears are carried off by means of a little tube which runs down into the nose from the inner corner of the eye. When the tears are formed so fast that they cannot all get away through this tube, they pass over the edge of the lower eyelid and flow down the cheek.

Muscles of the Eyes–By means of little muscles which are fastened to the eyeball, we are able to turn the eye in almost every direction.

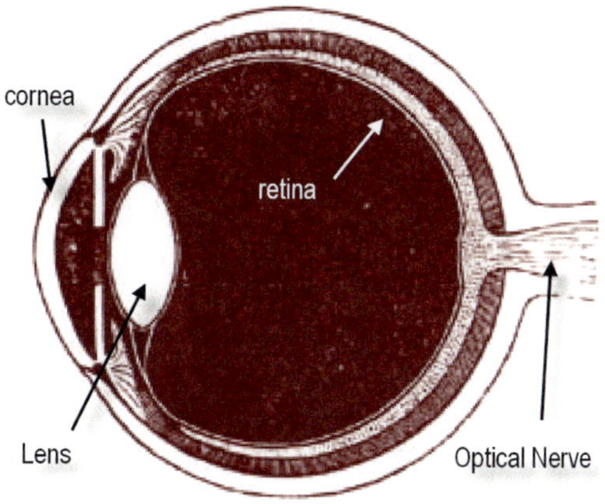

Inside of the Eye

Did you ever look through a spyglass or an opera-glass? If so, you know you must make the tube longer or shorter according as you look at things near by or far away. The eye also has to be changed a little when we look from near to distant objects. Look out of the window at a tree a long way off. Now place a lead pencil between the eyes and the tree. You can scarcely see the pencil while you look sharply at the tree, and if you look at the pencil you cannot see the tree distinctly.

There is a little muscle in the eye which makes the change needed to enable us to see objects close by as well as those which are farther away. When people grow old the little muscles cannot do this so well, and hence older people have to put on glasses to see objects near by, as in reading. Children should not try to wear older persons' glasses, as this is likely to injure their eyes.

How to Keep the Eyes Healthy–

(1) Never continue the use of the eyes at fine work, such as reading or fancy-work, after they have become very tired.

(2) Do not try to read or to use the eyes with a poor light–in the twilight, for instance, without a lamp to provide proper lighting.

(3.) In reading or studying, do not sit with the light from either a lamp or a window shining directly upon the face. Have the light come from behind and shine over the your shoulder if possible.

(4) Never expose the eyes to a sudden, bright light by looking at the sun or at a lamp on first awaking in the morning, or by passing quickly from a dark room into a lighted one.

(5) Do not read when lying down, or when riding in a car or train. The constant motion of the car or train causes your eyes to work harder.

(6) If any object gets into the eye have it removed as soon as possible.

(7) A great many persons hurt their eyes by using various kinds of eye-washes. Never use anything of this kind unless told to do so by a good physician.

How We Smell–If we wish to smell anything very strongly, we sniff or suddenly draw the air up through the nose. We do this to bring more air to the nerves of smell, which are placed at the upper part of the inside of the nose known as the nasal cavity. Dogs have a stronger sense of smell than people because dogs have more nerves of smell in their nasal cavity than do humans.

Smelling is a sort of feeling. The nerves of smell are so sensitive that they can discover things in the air which we cannot taste or see. A person may use their sense of smell to tell them whether things are good to eat or not. Things which have a pleasant smell are likely to be good for eating and not likely to make one sick.

People who do not use their sense of smell often are not able to smell so acutely. Many persons lose the sense of smell altogether from not caring for their body.

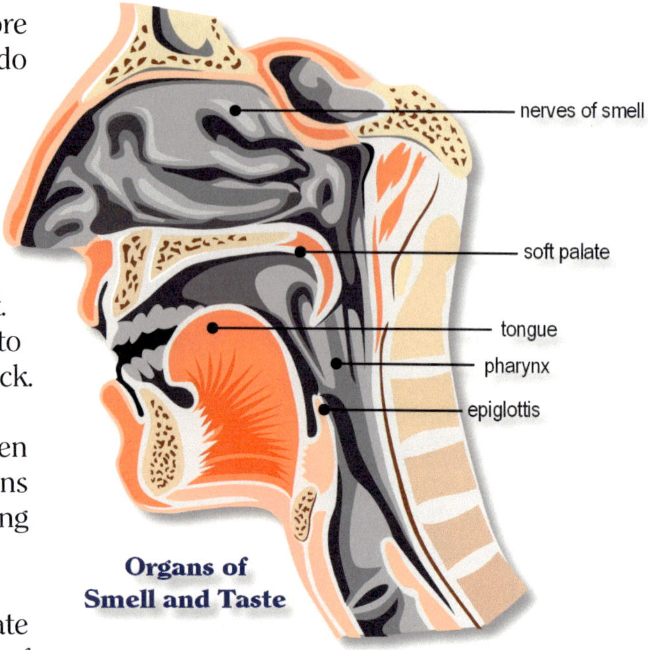

Organs of Smell and Taste

How We Taste–The tongue and the soft palate (pal´-uht) have very delicate nerves by means of which we taste. There are also nerves of taste in the epiglottis (ep-i-glot´-us) and pharynx (far´-inks). We cannot taste with the whole of the tongue. The very tip of the tongue has only nerves of touch or feeling.

The use of the sense of taste is to give us pleasure and to tell us whether different substances are healthful or injurious. Things which are poisonous and likely to make us sick almost always have an unpleasant taste as well as an unpleasant odor. Things which have a pleasant taste are usually harmless.

Bad Tastes–People sometimes learn to like things which have a very unpleasant taste. Pepper, mustard, pepper-sauce, and other hot sauces, alcohol, and tobacco are harmful substances of this sort. When used freely they injure the sense of taste so that it cannot detect and enjoy fine and delicate flavors. These substances, as we have elsewhere learned, also do the stomach harm and injure the nerves and other parts of the body.

The Sense of Touch–If you put your hand upon an object you can tell whether it is hard or soft, smooth or rough, and can learn whether it is round or square, or of some other shape. You are able to do this by means of the nerves of touch, which are found in the skin in all parts of the body. If you wished to know how an object feels, would you touch it with the elbow, or the knee, or the cheek? You will say, No. You would feel of it with the hand, and would touch it with the ends of the fingers. You can feel objects better with the ends of the fingers because there are more nerves of touch in the part of the skin covering the ends of the fingers than in most other parts of the body.

The sense of touch is more delicate in the tip of the tongue than in any other part. This is because it is necessary to use the sense of touch in the tongue to assist the sense of taste in finding out whether things are good to eat or not. The sense of touch is also very useful to us in many other ways. We hardly know how useful it really is until we are deprived of some of our other senses, as sight or hearing. In a blind man the sense of touch often becomes surprisingly sensitive.

Effects of Alcohol and Tobacco on the Special Senses–All the special senses–hearing, seeing, smelling, tasting, feeling–depend upon the brain and nerves. Whatever does harm to the brain and nerves must injure the special senses also. We have learned how alcohol and tobacco, and all other narcotics and stimulants, injure and sometimes destroy the brain cells and their nerve branches, and so we can understand that a person who uses these poisonous substances will, by so doing, injure the delicate organs with which he hears, sees, smells, etc.

Persons who use tobacco and strong drink sometimes become blind, because these poisons injure the nerves of sight. The ears are frequently injured by the use of tobacco. Smoking cigarettes and using snuff destroy the sense of smell. The poison of the tobacco paralyzes the nerves of taste so that they cannot detect flavors.

POINTS TO REMEMBER

1. We have five special senses: hearing, seeing, smelling, tasting, and feeling.

2. The ear is the organ of hearing, and has three parts, called the external ear, the middle ear, and the inner ear. The inner ear contains the nerve of hearing.

3. The middle ear is separated from the external ear by the tympanic membrane. The tympanic membrane is connected with the inner ear by a chain of bones.

4. Sounds cause the tympanic membrane to vibrate. The ear-bones convey the vibration from the tympanic membrane to the nerve of hearing.

5. To keep the ear healthy we must avoid meddling with it or putting things into it.

6. The eye is the organ of sight. The chief parts of the eye are the eyeball, the socket, and the eyelids.

7. In the eyeball are the pupil, the lens, and the retina.

8. The eyeball is moved in various directions by six small muscles.

9. The eye is moistened by tears from the tear gland.

10. When we look at an object the lens of the rods an cones on the retina make a picture that transmits to the nerve of sight, at the back part of the eyeball.

11. To keep the eyes healthy we should be careful not to tax them long at a time with fine work, or to use them in a poor light.

12. The nerves of smell are placed in the upper part of the inside of the nose.

13. Neglect of the body and disease can often destroy the sense of smell.

14. The nerves of taste are placed in the tongue, palate, epiglottis and pharynx.

15. Many things which we think we taste we really do not taste, but smell or feel.

16. Objects which have a pleasant taste are usually healthful, while those which have a bad taste are usually harmful.

17. Pepper, mustard, etc., as well as alcohol and tobacco, have an unpleasant taste, and are not healthful. If we use them we shall injure the nerves of taste as well as other parts of the body.

18. We feel objects by means of the sense of touch.

19. The sense of touch is most acute at the tip of the tongue and the ends of the fingers.

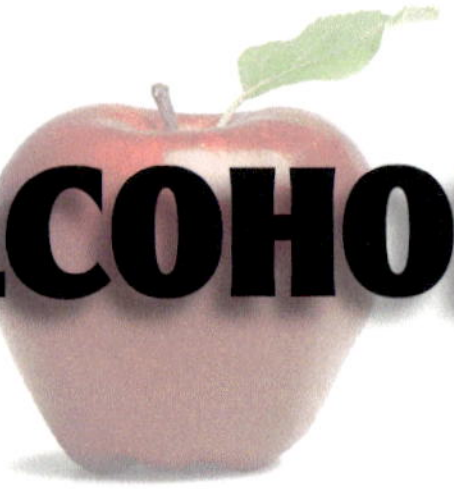

ALCOHOL

As we learned in the early part of our study of this subject, alcohol is produced by fermentation. It is afterwards separated from water and other substances by distillation. We will now learn a few more things about alcohol.

Alcohol Burns–If alcohol is placed in a kerosene lamp, it will burn much like kerosene oil. Indeed, it does not need a lamp to help it burn as does oil. If a few drops of alcohol are placed upon a plate, it may be lighted with a match, and will burn with a pale blue flame. Thus you see that alcohol is a sort of burning fluid.

The vapor of alcohol will burn also, and under some circumstances it will explode. On this account it is better not to try any experiments with it unless some older person is close by to direct you, so that no harm may be done. Alcohol is really a dangerous substance even though we do not take it as a drink.

We have told you that all fermented drinks contain alcohol. You will remember that wine, beer, ale, and cider are fermented drinks. We know that these drinks contain alcohol because the chemist can separate the alcohol from the water and other substances, and thus learn just how much alcohol each contains.

If we should remove all the alcohol from wine, no one would care to drink it. The same is true of beer and cider. It is very easy to remove the alcohol by the simple process of heating. This is the way the chemist separates it. The heat drives the alcohol off with the steam. If the heating is continued long enough, all the alcohol will be driven off. In China, people used to boil wine before drinking it. Perhaps this is one reason why Chinese were so seldom found drunken. In cooking, where wine or rum are used to flavor foods, the alcohol turns into a vapor as the food is cooked, and when the food is served, the alcohol is gone.

The Alcohol Breath–You have doubtless heard that a person who is under the influence of liquor may be known by his breath. His breath smells of alcohol. This is because his lungs are trying to remove the alcohol from his blood as fast as possible, so as to prevent injury to the blood corpuscles and the tissues of the body. It is the vapor of alcohol mixed with his breath that causes the odor. Alcohol alone is odorless.

You may have heard that sometimes men take such quantities of alcoholic drink that the breath becomes strong with the vapor of alcohol and takes fire when a light is brought near the mouth. These stories are probably not true.

Making Alcohol–Alcohol is made from the sweet juices of fruits by simply allowing them to ferment. Wine, as you know, is fermented grape juice. Cider is fermented apple juice. The strong alcoholic liquor obtained by distilling wine, cider, or any kind of fermented fruit juice, is known as brandy.

How Beer is Made–Beer is made from grain of some sort. The grain is first moistened and kept in a warm place for a few days until it begins to sprout. The young plant needs sugar for its food; and so while the grain is sprouting, the starch in the grain is changed into sugar by a curious kind of digestion. This, as you will remember, is the way in which the saliva acts upon starch. So far no very great harm has been done, only sprouted grain, though very sweet, is not so good to eat as grain which has not sprouted. Nature intends the sugar to be used as food for the little sproutlet; but the brewer wants it for another purpose, and he stops the growth of the plant by drying the grain in a hot room.

The next thing the brewer does is to grind the sprouted grain and soak it in water. The water dissolves out the sugar. Next he adds yeast to the sweet liquor and allows it to ferment, thus converting the sugar into alcohol. Potatoes are sometimes treated in a similar way.

By distilling beer, a strong liquor known as whiskey is obtained. Sometimes juniper berries are distilled with the beer. The liquor obtained is then called gin. In the West Indies, on the great sugar plantations, large quantities of liquor are made from the skimmings and cleanings of the vats in which the sweet juice of the sugar-cane is boiled down. These refuse matters are mixed with water and fermented, then distilled. This liquor is called rum.

Now you have learned enough about alcohol to know that it is not produced by plants in the same way that food is, but that it is the result of a sort of decay. In making alcohol, good food is destroyed and made into a substance which is not fit for food, and which produces a great amount of sickness and destroys many lives. Do you not think it a pity that such great quantities of good corn and other grains should be wasted in this way when they might be employed for a useful purpose?

The Alcohol Family–Scientists tell us that there are several different kinds of alcohol. Naphtha is a strong-smelling liquid sometimes used by painters to thin their paint and make it dry quickly. It does not have the same odor as alcohol, but it looks and acts very much like it. It will burn as alcohol does. It kills animals and plants. It will make a person drunk if he takes a sufficient quantity of it. Indeed, it is so like alcohol that it really is a kind of alcohol.

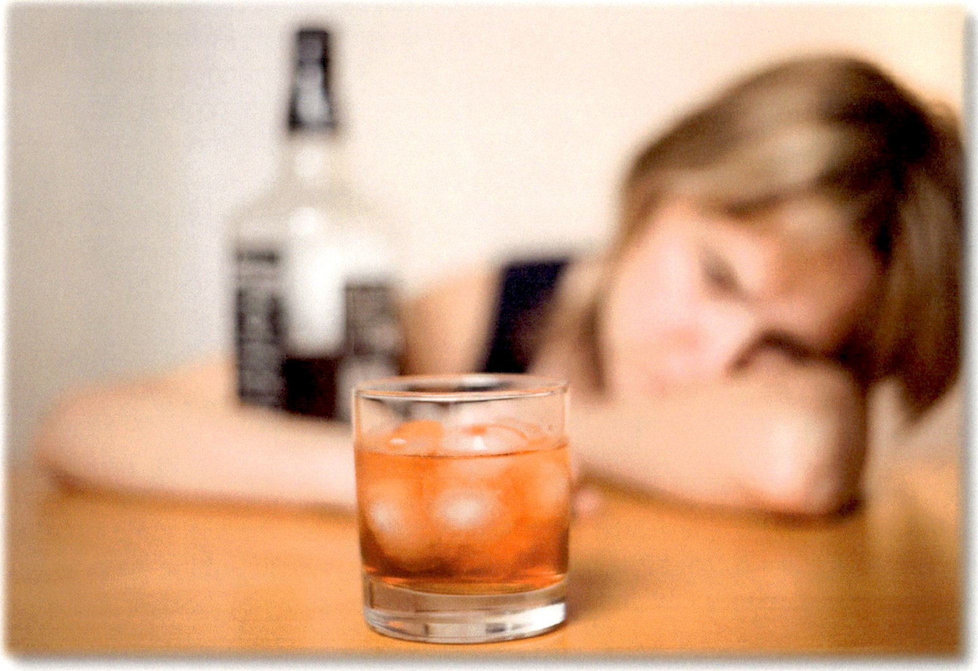

There are also other kinds of alcohol. Fusel-oil, a deadly poison, is an alcohol. A very small amount of this alcohol will make a person very drunk. Fusel-oil is found in bad whiskey. (All whiskey is bad, but some kinds are worse than others.) This is why such whiskey makes men so furiously drunk. It also causes speedy death in those who use it frequently. There are still other kinds of alcohol, some of which are even worse than fusel-oil. So you see this is a very bad family.

Like most other bad families, this alcohol family has many bad relations. You may have heard of phenol or carbolic acid, a powerful poison. This is one of the relatives of the alcohol family. Creosote is another poisonous substance closely related to alcohol. Ether and chloroform, by which people were once commonly made insensible during surgical operations, are also relatives of alcohol. They are, in fact, made from alcohol. These substances, although really useful, are very poisonous and dangerous. Do you not think it will be very wise and prudent for you to have nothing to do with alcohol in any form, even wine, beer, or cider, since it belongs to such a bad family and has so many bad relations?

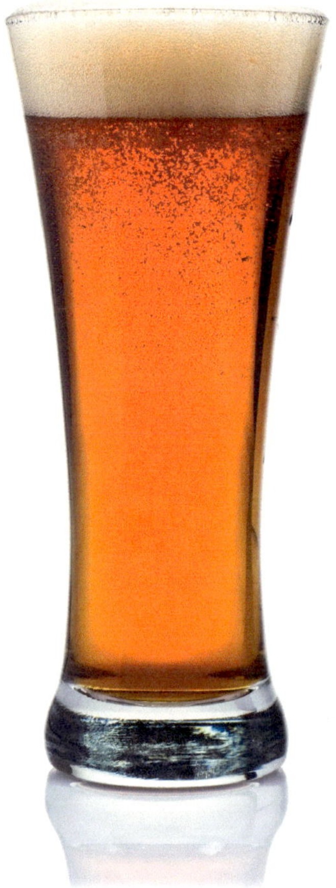

Some persons think that they will suffer no harm if they take only wine or beer, or perhaps hard cider. This is a great mistake. A person may get drunk on any of these drinks if a sufficient amount be taken. Besides, boys who use wine, beer, or cider, rarely fail to become fond of stronger liquors. A great many men who have died drunkards began with cider. Cider begins to ferment within a day or two after it is made, and becomes stronger in alcohol all the time for many months.

"Bitters"–There are other liquids not called "drinks" which contain alcohol. "Bitters" usually contain more alcohol than is found in ale or wine, and sometimes more than in the strongest whiskey. "Jamaica ginger" is almost pure alcohol. Hence, it is often as harmful for a person to use these medicines freely as to use alcoholic liquors in any other form.

Alcoholic liquors of all kinds are often adulterated. That is, they contain other poisons besides alcohol. In consequence of this, they may become even more harmful than when pure; but this does not make it safe to use even pure liquor. Alcohol is itself more harmful than the other drugs usually added in adulteration. It is important that you should know this, for many people think they will not suffer much harm from the use of alcohol if they are careful to obtain pure liquors.

Some Experiments–Do you remember what you have learned in previous lessons about the poisonous effects of alcohol? Do people ever die at once from its effects? Once a man made a bet that he could take five drinks of whiskey in five seconds. He dropped dead when he had swallowed the fourth glass. No one ever suffered such an effect from taking water or milk or any other good food or drink.

A man once made an experiment by mistake. He was carrying some alcohol across a lawn. He accidentally spilled some upon the grass. The next day he found the grass as dead and brown as though it had been scorched by fire.

A scientist once made a curious experiment. He took a little plant with three healthy green leaves, and shut it up under a glass jar where there was a teaspoonful of alcohol. The alcohol was in a dish by itself, so it did not touch the plant; but the vapor of the alcohol mixed with the air in the jar so that the plant had to breathe it. In less than half an hour he took the plant out. Its leaves were faded and somewhat shriveled The next morning it appeared to be dead. Do you suppose the odor of milk or meat, or of any good food, would affect a plant like that? Animals shut up with alcohol die in just the same way.

A Drunken Plant–How many of you remember about a curious plant that catches flies? Do you remember its name? What does the Venus flytrap do with the flies after it catches them? Do you say that it eats them? Really this is what it does, for it dissolves and absorbs them. In other words, it digests them. This is just what our stomachs do to the food we eat.

Two Experiments

PLEASE DO THESE WITH ADULT ASSISTANCE ONLY!

Experiment 1

Supplies
1 small piece of meat such as tender beefsteak
1 half cup of rubbing alcohol

Instructions
Place a piece of tender beefsteak in a saucer and cover it with alcohol. Put it away over night.

What Happens?
In the morning the beefsteak will be found to be shrunken, dried, and almost as tough as a piece of leather. This shows the effect of alcohol upon the tissues.

Experiment 2

Supplies
1 chicken egg
1 half glass of rubbing alcohol

Instructions
Break an egg into a half glassful of alcohol. Stir the egg and alcohol together for a few minutes.

What Happens?
Soon you will see that the egg begins to harden and look just as though it had been boiled.

A scientist thought that he would see what effect alcohol would have upon the digestion of a plant. So he put a fly-catching plant in a jar with some alcohol for just five minutes. The alcohol did not touch the plant, because the jar was only wet with the alcohol on the inside. When he took the plant out, he found that it could not catch flies, and that its digestion was spoiled so that it could not even digest very tender bits of meat which were placed on its leaves. The plant was drunk.

The scientist tried a great many experiments with various poisons, and found that the plants were affected in much the same way by ether and chloroform, and also by nicotine, the poisonous oil of tobacco. Sugar, milk, and other foods had no such effect. This does not look much as though alcohol would help digestion; does it?

Effects of Alcohol on Digestion–A very eminent English scientist made many experiments, many years ago, to ascertain positively about the effect of alcohol upon digestion. He concluded that alcohol, even in small doses, delays digestion. This is quite contrary to the belief of very many people, who suppose that wine, cider, or stronger liquors aid digestion. The use of alcohol in the form of beer or other alcoholic drinks is often a cause of serious disease of the stomach and other digestive organs.

Effects of Alcohol on Animal Heat–A large part of the food we eat is used in keeping our bodies warm. Most of the starch, sugar, and fat in our food serves the body as a sort of fuel. It is by this means that the body is kept always at about the same temperature, which is just a little less than one hundred degrees. This is why we need more food in very cold weather than in very warm weather.

When a person takes alcohol, it is found that instead of being made warmer by it, they are not so warm as before. They feel warmer, but if their temperature be measured by means of a thermometer placed in the mouth, it is found that they are really colder. The more alcohol a person takes the colder they become. If alcohol were good food would we expect this to be the case? It is probably true that the alcohol does make a little heat, but at the same time it causes us to lose much more heat than it makes. The outside of the body is not so warm as the inside. This is because the warm blood in the blood vessels of the skin is cooled more rapidly than the blood in the interior of the body. The effect of alcohol is to cause the blood vessels of the outside of the body to become much enlarged. This is why the face becomes flushed. A larger amount of warm blood is brought from the inside of the body to the outside, where it is cooled very rapidly; and thus the body loses heat, instead of gaining it, under the influence of alcohol. This is not true of any proper food substance.

Alcohol in the Polar Regions–Experience teaches the same thing as science respecting the effect of alcohol. Captain Ross, Dr. Kane, Captain Parry, Captain Hall, Lieutenant Greely, and many other famous explorers who have spent long months amid the ice and snow and intense cold of the countries near the North Pole, all say that alcohol does not warm a man when he is cold, and does not keep him from getting cold. Indeed, alcohol is considered so dangerous in these cold regions that no Arctic explorer at the present time could be induced to use it. Alcohol is a great deceiver, is it not? It makes a man think he is warmer, when he is really colder. Many men are frozen to death while drunk.

Alcohol in Hot Regions–Bruce, Livingstone, and Stanley, and all great African explorers, condemned the use of alcohol in that hot country as well as elsewhere. The Quechan (kwuh´-tsan) Indians, who live in Arizona and New Mexico, where the weather is sometimes much hotter than we ever know it here, made a law of their own against the use of liquor. If one of the tribe became drunk, he was severely punished. This law they made because of the evil effects of liquor which they noticed among the members of their tribe who used to become intoxicated. Do you not think that a very wise thing?

Sunstroke–Do you know what sunstroke is? If you do not, your parents or teacher will tell yow that persons exposed to the heat of the sun on a hot summer day are sometimes overcome by it. They become weak, giddy, or insensible, and not infrequently die. Scores of people are sometimes stricken down in a single day in some of our large cities. It may occur to you that if alcohol cools the body, it would be a good thing for a person to take to prevent or relieve an attack of sunstroke. On the contrary, it is found that those who use alcoholic drinks are much more liable to sunstroke than others. This is on account of the poisonous effects of the alcohol upon the nerves. No doctor would think of giving alcohol in any form to a man suffering with sunstroke.

The Effects of Alcohol on the Tissues–The two experiments described in this chapter show the effect of strong alcohol. The alcohol of alcoholic drinks has water and other things mixed with it, so that it does not act so quickly nor so severely as pure alcohol; but the effect is essentially the same in character. It is partly in this way that the brain, nerves, muscles, and other tissues of drinking men and women become diseased.

Eminent physicians tell us that a large share of the unfortunate persons who are shut up in psychiatric hospitals are brought there by alcohol. Is it not a dreadful thing that one's mind should be thus ruined by a useless and harmful practice?

POINTS TO REMEMBER

1. Alcohol is produced by fermentation, and obtained by distillation. It will burn like kerosene oil and other burning fluids.

2. The vapor of alcohol will burn and will sometimes explode.

3. Alcohol may be separated from beer and other fermented liquids by boiling.

4. Brandy is distilled from fermented fruit juice, whiskey and gin from beer or fermented grains, rum from fermented molasses.

5. Alcohol is the result of a sort of decay, and much good food is destroyed in producing it.

6. Besides ordinary alcohol, there are several other kinds. Naphtha and fusel-oil are alcohols.

7. All the members of the alcohol family are poisons; all will burn, and all will intoxicate. The alcohol family have several bad relations, among which are phenol, ether, and chloroform.

8. Cider, beer, and wine are harmful and dangerous as well as strong liquors. "Bitters" often contain as much alcohol as the strongest liquors, and sometimes more.

9. Alcoholic liquors are sometimes adulterated, but they usually contain no poison worse than alcohol. Pure alcohol is scarcely less dangerous than that which is adulterated.

10. Death sometimes occurs almost instantly from taking strong liquors.

11. Alcohol will kill grass and other plants, if poured upon them or about their roots.

12. The vapor of alcohol will kill plants; also plants become intoxicated by breathing the vapor of alcohol.

13. Alcohol, even in small quantities, hinders digestion.

14. Alcohol causes the body to lose heat so rapidly that it becomes cooler instead of warmer.

15. The danger of freezing to death when exposed to extreme cold is greatly increased by taking alcohol.

16. Stanley, and other African explorers, say that it is dangerous to use alcoholic drinks in hot climates.

17. In very hot weather, persons who use alcoholic drinks are more subject to sunstroke than those who do not.

18. Beefsteak soaked in alcohol becomes tough like leather. An egg placed in alcohol is hardened as though it had been boiled.

19. The effect of alcohol upon the brain, nerves, and other tissues of the body is much the same as upon the beefsteak and the egg.

QUESTIONS for REVIEW

THE HOUSE WE LIVE IN–What is the body like? Does the body resemble anything else besides a house? How is it like a machine? Name the different parts of the body. What is anatomy? physiology? hygiene?

AN OVERVIEW OF THE BODY–What are the main parts of the body? Name the different parts of the head; of the trunk; of each arm; of each leg. What covers the body?

THE INSIDE OF THE BODY–What is the name of the framework of the body? What is the skull? How is the spinal column formed? Name the two cavities of the trunk. What does the chest contain? the abdomen?

OUR FOODS–Of what are our bodies made? What are foods? Where do we get our foods? Name some animal foods; some vegetable foods. What are poisons?

UNHEALTHFUL FOODS–Is the flesh of diseased animals good for food? What can you say about unripe, stale, or moldy foods? What is adulteration of foods? What foods are most likely to be adulterated? Are pepper, mustard, and other condiments proper foods? What about tobacco? What is the effect of tobacco upon children?

OUR DRINKS–What is the only thing that will satisfy thirst? Why do we need water? How does water sometimes become impure? What is the effect of using impure water? What are the properties of good water? Are caffeinated tea and coffee good drinks? How is alcohol made? Give familiar examples of fermentation. How are pure alcohol and strong liquors made? Is alcohol a food? Why do you think it is a poison? Do you think moderate drinking is healthful?

HOW WE DIGEST–What is digestion? What is the digestive tube? Name the different digestive organs. How many sets of teeth has a person in his lifetime? How many teeth in each set? How many pairs of salivary glands? What do they form? What is the gullet or esophagus? Describe the stomach. What is the gastric fluid? How long is the intestinal canal? What fluid is formed in the intestines? Where is the liver found, and how large is it? What does the liver produce? What is the gall bladder, and what is its use? What does the liver do besides producing bile? What and where is the pancreas? What does the pancreas do? Where is the spleen? How many important organs of digestion are there? How many digestive fluids?

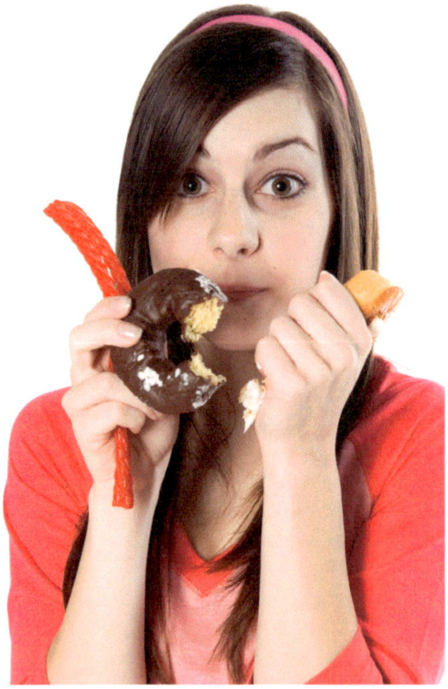

DIGESTING A MOUTHFUL–Name the different processes of digestion [mastication, action of saliva, swallowing, action of stomach and gastric fluid, action of bile, action of pancreatic fluid, action of intestines and intestinal fluid, absorption, liver digestion]. Describe the digestion of a mouthful of bread. Where is the food taken after it has been absorbed? What are the lacteals? What is the thoracic duct?

BAD HABITS IN EATING–What is indigestion? Mention some of the causes of indigestion. How does eating too fast cause indigestion? Eating too much? too frequently? Irregularly? when tired? How do caffeinated tea and coffee impair digestion? Why is it harmful to use iced foods and drinks? Why should we not eat pepper and other hot and irritating things? How should the teeth be cared for? How does tobacco-using affect the stomach? What dreadful disease is sometimes caused by tobacco? How does alcohol affect the gastric fluid? the stomach? the liver?

A DROP OF BLOOD–What does the blood contain? How many kinds of blood cells are there? What work is done for the body by each kind of cells?

WHY THE HEART BEATS–Where is the heart? Why does the heart beat? How many chambers has the heart? What are the blood vessels? How many kinds of blood vessels are there? Name them. What is the difference between venous blood and arterial blood? What change occurs in the blood in the lungs? What is the pulse? How much work does the heart do every twenty-four hours? What are the lymphatics? What do they contain, and what is their purpose? What are lymphatic glands?

A HEALTHY HEART and BLOOD–Name some things likely to injure the heart or the blood. What is the effect of violent exercise? of bad air? of bad food? of loss of sleep? of violent anger? What can you say about clothing? What is the effect of alcohol upon the blood? the heart? the bodily heat? What is the effect of tobacco upon the heart? the pulse? the blood? What is the effect of tea and coffee upon the heart? What is a cold? In a case of bleeding from a wound, how can you tell whether a vein or an artery is cut? How would you stop the bleeding from an artery? from a vein? How would you stop nose-bleed?

WHY and HOW WE BREATHE–What happens to a lighted candle if shut up in a small, close place? to a mouse? Why is air so necessary for a burning candle and for animals? How is the heat of our bodies produced? Name the principal organs of breathing. Describe each. How do we use the lungs in breathing? How much air will a man's lungs hold? How much air do we use with each breath? What poisonous substance does the air which we breathe out contain? Will a candle burn in air which has been breathed? What happens to animals placed in such air? What change takes place in the blood as it passes through the lungs? How do plants purify the air?

KEEPING YOUR LUNGS HEALTHY–What is the thing most necessary to preserve life? Name some of the ways in which the blood becomes impure. Why is bad-smelling air dangerous to health? What are germs? Why are some diseases contagious? Name some such diseases. What should be done with a person who has a contagious disease? What is the effect of the breath upon the air? How much air is poisoned and made unfit to breathe by each breath? How much air do we spoil every minute? every hour? How much pure air does each person need every minute? every hour? How do we get fresh air into our houses? Why are windows and doors not good means of ventilating in cold weather? How should a room be ventilated? How should we use the lungs in breathing? What about the clothing in reference to the lungs? Why is it injurious to breathe habitually through the mouth? What is the effect of alcohol upon the lungs? What is the effect of tobacco-using upon the throat and nose?

THE SKIN and WHAT IT DOES–How many layers in the skin? What is each called? To what is the color of the skin due? What glands are found in the dermis? What are the nails and what is their purpose? How does the hair grow? Name the different uses of the skin?

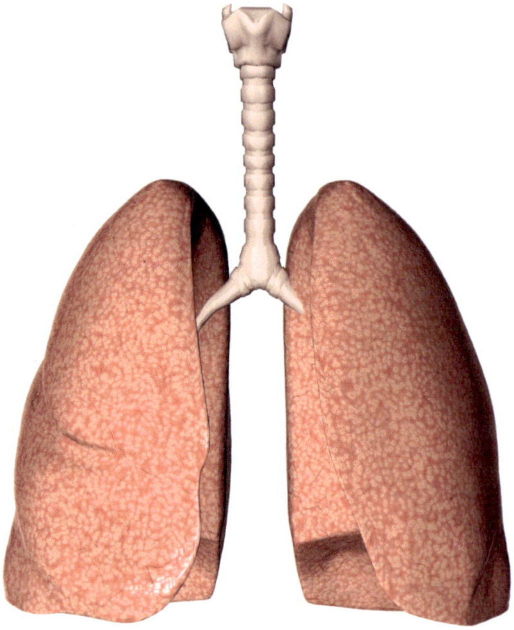

HOW TO CARE FOR THE SKIN–What happened to the little boy who was covered with gold leaf? Why did he die? What is the effect of neglecting to keep the skin clean? What is the effect of wearing too much clothing and living in rooms which are too warm? How should the hair be cared for? the nails? What is the effect of alcohol, tobacco, and other narcotics upon the skin?

THE KIDNEYS and THEIR WORK–What is the work of the kidneys? How may we keep these organs healthy? What is the effect of alcohol upon the kidneys?

OUR BONES and THEIR USES–How many bones in the body? What are the bones called when taken all together? Name the principal parts of the skeleton. Name the bones of the trunk, of the arms, of the legs. What are the uses of the bones? What is a joint? What is cartilage? By what are the bones held together? Of what are the bones largely composed?

KEEPING YOUR BONES HEALTHY–What sort of bread is best for the bones? Why? What are the effects of sitting or lying in bad positions? Of wearing tight or poorly-fitting clothing? Of tight or high-heeled shoes? What injuries are likely to happen to the bones and joints by accident or rough play?

MUSCLES and HOW WE USE THEM–How many muscles in the body? Of what are the muscles composed? How are many of the muscles connected to the bones? To what are all bodily movements due? How do the muscles act? What causes the muscles to act? Do all muscles act only when we will to have them act?

KEEPING MUSCLES HEALTHY–What makes the right arm of the shot put or discus thrower stronger than the left one? How should exercise be taken? Mention some things in relation to the use of the muscles which we ought not to do, and state the reasons why. What is the effect of alcohol upon the muscles? of tobacco? of caffeinated tea and coffee?

HOW WE FEEL and THINK–With what part of the body do we think? How many brains does a man have? How is each brain divided? Of what is the brain largely composed? Where do the nerves begin? What is the spinal cord? Why does it cause pain to prick the finger? Name some of the different kinds of nerves of feeling? Name some of the different kinds of work controlled by the nerves of work. Of what use to the body are the brain and nerves? How does the brain use the nerves? Of what use is the large brain? What does the little brain do? Of what use is the spinal cord?

A HEALTHY BRAIN and NERVES–Mention some things which we need to do to keep the brain and nerves healthy. Mention some things which we ought not to do.

POISONING THE BRAIN and NERVES–What is the effect of alcohol upon the brain and nerves? Does alcohol produce real strength? Does it produce real warmth? Does alcohol make people better or worse? What is the effect of tobacco upon the brain and nerves? Does the use of tobacco lead to other evil habits? What about the effect of opium and other narcotics?

HOW WE HEAR, TASTE, SMELL–How many senses have we? What is the ear? Name the three parts of the ear. How do we hear? How should we treat the ear?

Name the principal parts of the eye? What are found in the eyeball? How is the eyeball moved in the socket? How is the eye moistened? Of what use is the lens of the eye? Of what use is the pupil of the eye? How may we preserve the eyesight?

Where are the nerves of smell located? Of what use is the sense of smell?

Where are the nerves of taste found? How is the sense of taste sometimes injured or lost? What do we detect with the sense of taste? Of what use to us is the sense of taste?

With what sense do we feel objects? In what parts of the body is this sense most delicate? Upon what do all the special senses depend? Does anything that injures the brain and nerves also injure the special senses? What is the effect of alcohol and tobacco upon the sense of sight? How is the hearing affected by tobacco-using? The sense of smell? The sense of taste?

ALCOHOL–How is alcohol produced? In what respect is alcohol like kerosene oil? Is alcohol a dangerous thing even if we do not drink it? ? Can you tell by the odor of his breath when a person has been drinking? Why? From what is brandy made? How are whiskey, gin, and rum made? Is alcohol a result of growth, like fruits and grains, or of decay? Is there more than one kind of alcohol? Mention some of the members of the alcohol family. In what ways are the members of this family alike? Name some of the bad relations. Are cider and beer, as well as whiskey, dangerous? Why? Mention some other things, besides drinks, which contain alcohol. Are alcoholic drinks adulterated? Is pure alcohol safe? Is instant death ever produced by alcohol? Will alcohol kill plants? Describe the experiment which proved this. Can plants be made drunk by alcohol? Describe the experiment which proves this. What has been proven concerning the influence of alcohol upon digestion? How are our bodies kept warm? Explain how alcohol makes the body cooler? Do Arctic explorers use alcohol? Why not? Does the use of alcohol prevent sunstroke? What did Stanley and Livingstone say about the use of alcohol in Africa? What is the effect of using alcohol upon meat and eggs? What is the effect of alcohol upon the brain and other tissues of the body? Does alcohol cause insanity and other diseases of the brain and nerves?

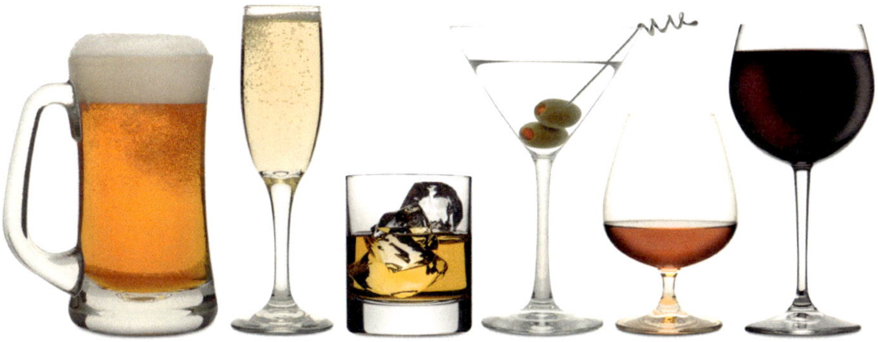

ABOUT DR. JOHN HARVEY KELLOGG

(February 26, 1852 - December 14, 1943)

John Harvey Kellogg's contributions to the science of health and nutrition far exceed the invention for which he is best known: corn flake cereal. John was born in Tyrone, Michigan in 1852, the son of John Preston Kellogg and his second wife, Anne Jeanette Stanley. The Kellogg family moved to Battle Creek, Michigan, when John was four years old. There his father set up a broom factory.

A Christian family belonging to the newly-formed Seventh-day Adventist Church, the Kelloggs participated actively in the growing church's activities. John's parents contributed money toward the building of the Battle Creek's Western Health Reform Institute, founded to promote the Adventist's health message by providing a retreat where people could learn about proper nutrition, how to treat and prevent common illness, and how to care for the health of the body. John was befriended by James and Ellen White, two leaders of the Seventh-day Adventist movement who were also instrumental in starting the Western Health Reform Institute. James and Ellen saw in John unique talents, and sponsored John's education at New York University Medical College at Bellevue Hospital. There John received training as a physician and surgeon, then upon his graduation returned to Battle Creek where he became at age 24 the medical director of the Western Health Reform Institute.

Shortly after John Kellogg M.D. took on leadership of the Institute it had twenty patients. John changed the name to Battle Creek Sanitarium--*sanitarium* a word he created to describe a place where people would learn to stay well. In time, John's charismatic personality and leadership helped attract people from around the world to Battle Creek Sanitarium. The San, as it was called, became Kellogg's laboratory for his "Battle Creek Idea" that good health and fitness result from good diet, exercise, correct posture, fresh air and proper rest. At its high point, The San kept a staff of approximately 1,800 workers. In 1927, its fiftieth year, The San served 4,000 patients. The rich and famous flocked to Battle Creek, often making annual trips of several weeks. Among the celebrities to receive care at The San were President William Taft, automaker Henry Ford, and famous airplane pilot Amelia Earhart. Here they were pampered in elegant surroundings while their bodies were

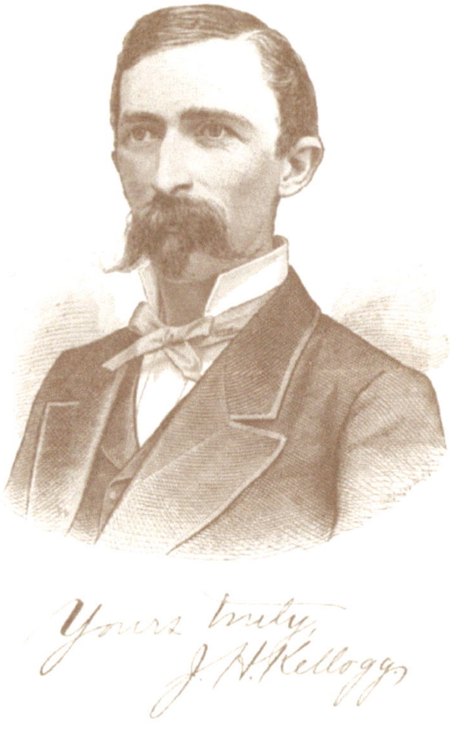

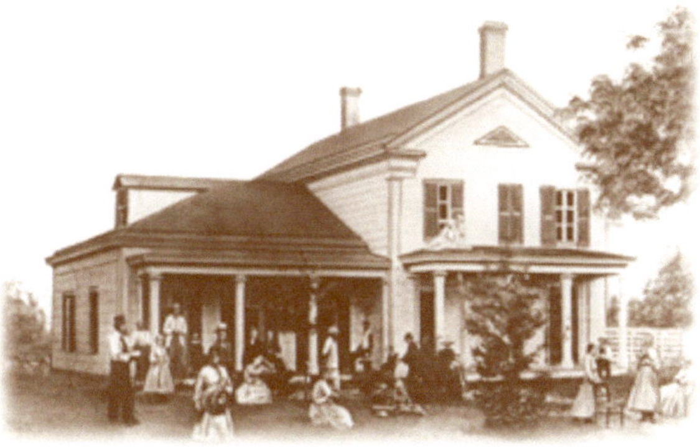

Western Health Reform Institute

restored to health with a nutritious diet and scientifically planned exercise.

In 1877, only a year after joining The San, Dr. Kellogg invented The San's first health food--a breakfast cereal called "granola." He also developed a coffee substitute made from grains. Together with his brother William, who worked as The San's bookkeeper, the corn flake launched a breakfast food industry for which Battle Creek, Michigan, is still known today. In all, Dr. Kellogg invented some 80 grain and nut products. In 1901, Dr. Kellogg and William launched the Sanitas Food Company, which later became the Kellogg Food Company.

Dr. Kellogg and William did not always see eye-to-eye. In 1920 their differences led to Dr. Kellogg and William parting ways, leaving the Kellogg Food Company and the rights to the Kellogg brand name to William.

Dr. Kellogg dedicated much of his adult life to education to improve his medical knowledge and surgical skills. He made several trips to Europe to study medicine, surgery and physiology with leading European medical figures. He was a fellow of the leading medical societies, including the American Association for the Advancement of Science, American College of Surgeons and the American Medical Association.

He was a very successful surgeon, performing some 22,000 operations during his 67 year career. He accepted no pay for his work with The San or for any of his surgeries. His entire income came from royalties from the nearly 50 books and medical writings published during his long career. Dr. Kellogg wrote primarily about "biologic living," constantly working to educate the public and other doctors about his health reform ideas. He also introduced to medical science several new techniques, primarily in abdominal surgery.

Dr. Kellogg married Ella Ervilla Eaton of Alfred Center, New York, on February 22, 1879. They did not have any children of their own, but raised over forty children, legally adopting seven before Ella died in 1920.

Dr. Kellogg's legacy includes several teachings and discoveries that are still widely respected today, such as those in this book. However, as he aged, he developed many controversial and poorly founded ideas that have stained his reputation. At the age of seventy-eight, Kellogg moved to Florida and renovated the Country Club Hotel–which was donated by a previous patron, the pioneer aircraft manufacturer Glenn Curtiss–and opened the Miami-Battle Creek Sanitarium, a 100-bed establishment, which ran at capacity for his remaining thirteen years of life.

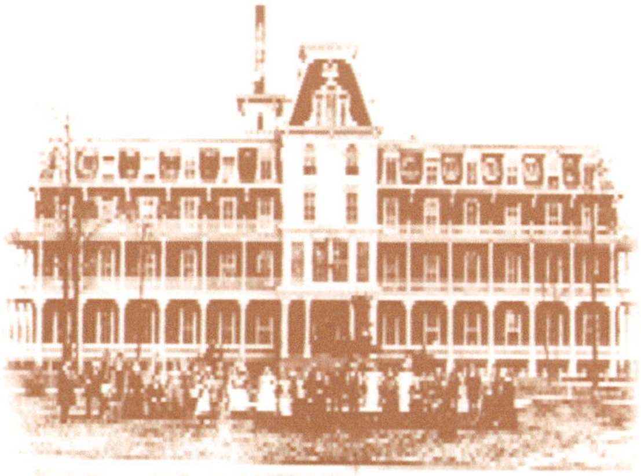

Battle Creek Sanitarium 1878

Enhance your child's learning with the companion workbook!

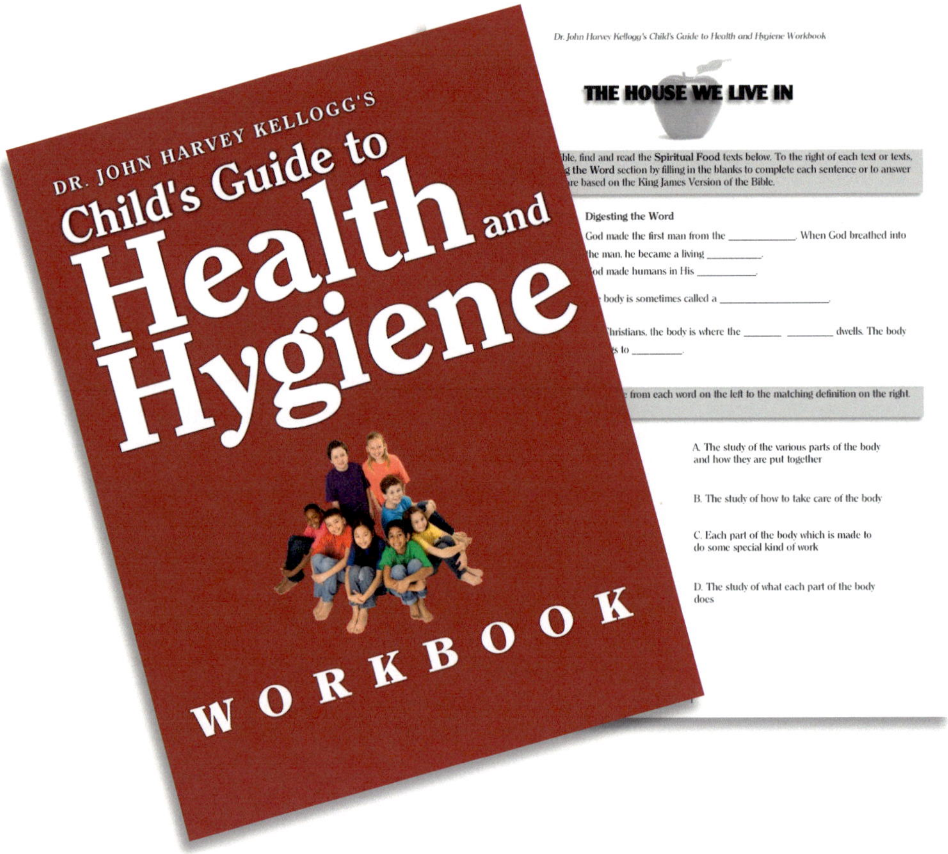

Available at
http://Kellogg.MustardSeedImprints.com

QUICK ORDER FORM

Internet Orders: http://kellogg.MustardSeedImprints.com
E-mail Orders: orders@MustardSeedImprints.com
Postal Orders: Mustard Seed Imprints, PO Box 1211, Clackamas, OR 97015

Name: ____

Mailing Address: ________________________________

City: ___________________________ **State:**____________ **ZIP:** ______________

Telephone: ______________________ **Email:** ______________________________

Quantity	Title	Cost	Total (quantity x cost)
	DR. JOHN HARVEY KELLOGG'S CHILD'S GUIDE TO HEALTH AND HYGIENE	$14.95	
	U.S. Media Mail Shipping *	$3.50	
		Total Enclosed	

***Please contact us by e-mail or purchase on our website for international or express shipping.**

Visit KidsBibleInfo.com
Big Answers for Little People

Made in United States
Troutdale, OR
04/15/2026

48531167R00057